THE LEMONG -RASS

The benefits of lemongrass

BY EDDIE PARKER

Contents

Abstract

Lemongrass is the strongest natural stimulant and adaptogen that relieves both physical and mental fatigue, significantly increasing the strength of the body. It is not for nothing that lemongrass has been a recognized medicine of Chinese healers for thousands of years - dynasties changed, and emperors continued to prolong their life and youth with its help.

In this book you will find various methods of disease prevention and treatment with lemongrass, ways to improve the overall health of the body with lemongrass, get acquainted with many recipes for using lemongrass to enhance physical and mental performance, as well as tips for growing lemongrass in the garden.

This publication is not a medical textbook. All treatment procedures must be agreed with the attending physician.

Tatyana Litvinova

The great medicine of Chinese emperors for 1000 diseases. Lemongrass: how to be treated and how to grow

Foreword "Berry with five tastes", with the help of whichthe emperors of ancient China extended their lives

About twelve years ago, I discovered an amazing medicine - Chinese magnolia vine. By this time, I was pretty exhausted by vegetative-vascular dystonia and frequent pressure drops, which brought me to physical exhaustion: dizziness, unsteadiness when walking, tinnitus, my forehead tightens as if with a mesh, sometimes there is not enough air, a feeling that the lungs when inhaling to the end cannot be filled. Plus mental symptoms: insomnia, anxiety, irritability, unmotivated anxiety. This went on for several months, the advice of doctors did not help. Lemongrass saved me! At a neighbor's dacha, these beautiful bushes grew - creepers with bright orange fruits, and the neighbor gave me berries and told me how to make tincture, infusion and decoction from them and how to treat them. At first, I just chewed berries every morning for three weeks - 4 berries each. Gradually, the symptoms of the disease began to disappear. Then - on the advice of those who had known lemongrass for a long time - she began to make infusions and decoctions not only from berries, but also from leaves and shoots of lemongrass. Six months later, I cautiously stated that the symptoms of my illness seemed to have gone completely. I was not mistaken, and lemongrass became my constant friend and still gives me full-fledged vital energy. During the year I use it in courses - either tea from the leaves, then a spring decoction from young twigs, then fresh berries, then dry, then jam from berries, then juice. In late summer and early autumn, orange-red schisandra berries can be added to any tea. And bouquets of lemongrass branches purify the air in the house! For the winter, you can always dry the leaves, and twigs, and berries. who has known lemongrass for a long time - began to make infusions and decoctions not only from berries, but also from leaves and shoots of lemongrass. Six months later, I cautiously stated that the symptoms of my illness seemed to have gone completely. I was not mistaken, and lemongrass became my constant friend and still gives me full-fledged vital energy. During the year I use it in courses - either tea from the leaves, then a spring decoction from young twigs, then fresh berries, then dry, then jam from berries, then juice. In late summer and early autumn, orange-red schisandra berries can be added to any tea. And bouquets of lemongrass branches purify the air in the house! For the winter, you can always dry the leaves, and twigs, and berries. who has known lemongrass for a long time - began to make infusions and decoctions not only from berries, but also from leaves and shoots of lemongrass. Six months later, I cautiously stated that the symptoms of my illness seemed to have gone completely. I was not mistaken, and lemongrass became my constant friend and still gives me full-fledged vital energy. During the year I use it in courses - either tea from the leaves, then a spring decoction from young twigs, then fresh berries, then dry, then jam from berries, then juice. In late summer and early autumn, orange-red schisandra berries can be added to any tea. And bouquets of lemongrass branches purify the air in the house! For the winter, you can always dry the leaves, and twigs, and berries. and lemongrass became my constant friend and still gives me full-fledged vital energy. During the year I use it in courses - either tea from the leaves, then a spring decoction from young twigs, then fresh berries, then dry, then jam from berries, then juice. In late summer and early autumn, orange-red schisandra berries can be added to any tea. And bouquets of lemongrass branches purify the air in the house! For the winter, you can always dry the leaves, and twigs, and berries. and lemongrass became my constant friend and still gives me full-fledged vital energy. During the year I use it in courses - either tea from the leaves, then a spring decoction from young twigs, then fresh berries, then dry, then jam from berries, then juice. In late summer and early autumn, orange-red schisandra berries can be added to any tea. And bouquets of lemongrass branches purify the air in the house! For the winter, you can always dry the leaves, and twigs, and berries.

I planted this miracle in my dacha - bushes bloom beautifully, and lemongrass ripens beautifully in autumn! And there are enough berries for my whole family, for friends and relatives. And berries, and branches, and bark, and leaves, and seeds - because lemongrass is healing all: from top to toe! Healer, energy drinker, adaptogen is always at hand! It turned out that growing lemongrass is not a problem, it does not require too much special care. For some reason, in central Russia, this taiga doctor is not very common, which is a pity - lemongrass grows without problems in our region. I heard stories from friends of summer residents who also have this amazing plant: from what only lemongrass saved! And he helped to survive stress, and long-distance flights with a change in time zones and climate, students to pass exams after sleepless nights, grandparents to correct their stomachs and eyesight! And our long trips! When you have to travel 800 km to relatives, spend a day there and immediately go back - for two nights my husband is driving, only lemongrass saves him. In addition, the husband corrected his eyesight with the help of a medicinal plant - when his eyesight began to deteriorate with age, he began to chew 1-2 leaves of lemongrass in the morning, as a result, glasses prescribed by an ophthalmologist were not needed. The same leaves and fatigue warn, I checked for myself: working in the country on the weekend does not tire as much as before, and any other work does, too. Leaves to tastebitter, if chewed for several minutes, the gruel in the mouth will resemble something like jelly.

Of course, having planted five seedlings of lemongrass (now I have a dozen of these vines), I immediately rushed to collect everything I could find about the magnificent bush: recipes for using lemongrass for various diseases, recipes for increasing vitality and immunity, recipes for preventing common ailments. It turned out that Chinese magnolia vine is one of the most ancient plants on the planet, a real relic, and the ancient Chinese have long used lemongrass as a powerful healing, tonic, and strength-giving remedy.

The emperors of ancient China extended their youth and life thanks to the great healing potential of the red-orange berry. It is not for nothing that lemongrass has long been called in China the court plant of Chinese emperors.

My seedlings have turned into large vines, and I am still updating my knowledge about the healing properties of lemongrass. Perhaps the information I have collected about the amazing effect of the berries of life, as the ancient Chinese called lemongrass, on the human body will help all those who are now reading this book.

Schisandra chinensis is not just a beautiful orange-red berry. This is an amazing natural remedy with amazing healing properties. Lemongrass treats and prevents a huge number of diseases. Due to the excellent composition of substances,located in lemongrass, this plant so powerfully stimulates, strengthens, heals, tones our body that the diseases accumulated in it

- recede, and new ones - do not arise. It is the strongest natural stimulant and adaptogen that relieves both physical and mental fatigue, increases the strength of the body tenfold and allows us not only not to get sick in extreme conditions, but to quickly and efficiently adapt to them. Everything is useful in this ancient creeper - and berries, and leaves, and flowers, and stems, and seeds, and bark, and roots. But the first in terms of healing are the seeds. If roots, stemor grind a lemongrass berry, you can clearly hear the smell of lemon, hence the Russian name.

Back in the fifth century BC, the Chinese called lemongrass - "wu-wei-tzu" - a fruit with five tastes. The peel of the berries has a sweet taste, the pulp is sour, the seeds of lemongrass are bitter and burning, in total these tastes give the berry a general salty tart taste, and the leaves and stems of the plant have a delicate lemon aroma. And the number five is not accidental. The fact is that in the treatment of diseases and the manufacture of medicines by Chinese healers, the system of interaction between man and the Universe was taken into account, and in this system an important role belonged to magic numbers, including the number five: the doctrine of the five elements, the five categories of human character, the five temperaments, about the five main plants for proper nutrition, etc. And medicines were prepared in such a way that they correctly combined the five tastes.

There are many legends and tales about the powerful healing power of lemongrass. The image of a hungry and exhausted Chinese youth who got entangled in the tenacious lianas of lemongrass and lost consciousness, but completely regained his strength by eating a bunch bright berries - this is not at all a legendary ancient metaphor, but the most real reality. Lemongrass - in terms of its powerful usefulness - in oriental medicine is in second place after ginseng, in China in the old days it was even included in the list of taxes that were necessarily paid to the emperor. And the hunters of the Far East, where lemongrass still, fortunately, grows wild to this day, going to the taiga, ate a handful of healing berries and could follow the trail of the beast all day without feeling exhausting fatigue. In addition, at night they began to see better. This property of lemongrass was used during the Great Patriotic WarSoviet pilots: before night flights, they used lemongrass preparations as a remedy that drove away sleep and sharpened vision in the dark.

Modern scientists have found that 100 g of schisandra berries contain a daily dose of vitamin C, a lot of vitamin P, beta-carotene, vitamin E, pectins, minerals, essential oils, a lot of citric acid, and in terms of sugar content (20%), schisandra berries comparable to grapes. Schisandra is especially valued for substances called lignans. One of them - schizandrin - has an exciting effect on the nervous system, about the same as a brazil nut.

"cola". Thanks to lignans, lemongrass enhances physical and mental activity, the body's resistance to any negative factors, stimulates the heart and blood vessels, and strengthens the entire body.

The founder of medicinal gardening, Professor L. I. Vigorov, wrote: "Schisandra should be remembered in case of loss of strength and reduced efficiency, depression, the need to ensure high concentration when performing a particularly important task or especially hard work."

In addition to the use of lemongrass as a restorative and Schizandra has long been used in Chinese and Korean medicine for the prevention and treatment of many diseases.

Lemongrass will help with bronchitis, pneumonia, bronchial

asthma, inflammation of the kidneys and urinary incontinence, cardiovascular problems of a functional nature and drowsiness, diseases of the stomach and intestines, motion sickness and diarrhea, diabetes mellitus and impotence. Lemongrass is necessary for hypotension and vision problems, for asthenia and asthenic depression. This plant relieves any fatigue, regulates the acidity of gastric juice, is an assistant to the main medicines for tuberculosis, fights eczema and skin inflammation, reduces the risk of getting the flu several times. Lemongrass will cope with toxicosis during pregnancy and menopausal disorders, help the body adapt to extreme external conditions and increase visual acuity.

This is a very powerful remedy, so the prevention and treatment of lemongrass should be dealt with strictly scheduled courses and under the supervision of a doctor! You can not resort to this natural medicine for hypertension, nervous excitement and insomnia, stomach ulcers, acute cardiac disorders.

But many diseases can be prevented or significantly mitigated, if they have already arisen, if you use lemongrass correctly. And this book will teach you how to use natural medicine correctly. Together with Lemongrass you can:

Increase the body's defense against any adverse external

influences.

Keep your immune system strong.

Quickly restore strength after physical and mental stress.

Treat respiratory diseases and colds.

Help the heart and blood vessels.

Heal the gastrointestinal tract and kidneys.

Cope with fatigue, depression and drowsiness.

Fight diabetes.

Contribute to the long-term preservation of women's and men's health.

Improve eyesight.

Keep your skin healthy and beautiful.

In this book, I tried to collect the best recipes and tips forthe use of lemongrass as a universal and powerful

energy means to maintain excellent health. Purpose of the book

- to show how a magnificent plant works for healing, rejuvenation and toning the body, and take a number of steps along with lemongrass to well-being.

Chapter 1 Healer, stimulant, tonic

Lemongrass - not the most familiarplant for central Russia. And for Ancient China, lemongrass was nothing less than an ordinary miracle. Ordinary, because he grew up there in the wild (as in our Far East), and miraculously - because he treated almost all ailments and bestowed not only emperors, but also mere mortals with youth and long life.

About the amazing longevity of the rulers of China, not only legends tell, but also documents. And none of the various legendary or historical testimonies is complete without the mention of lemongrass. Unique, sung by ancient Chinese poets (among them wereemperors!) five-tasting bright berries with their sour, bitter, sweet, spicy and salty notes prolonged the life of many rulers of the Celestial Empire.

Legendary emperor Fu-hsi, inventoracupuncturist, who lived almost 5 thousand years ago, ruled his subjects for 15 years, Shen-nong, who had extensive knowledge in medicine, taught the Chinese how to cultivate land - 140 years, and the universally revered Huangdi, who distinguished himself by creating sciences and crafts - 10 years . Lemongrass not only extended their life, but also served as a kind of panacea for diseases.

As the ancient Chinese testimonies mention,lemongrass neverwas translated into the diet of long-lived emperors, therefore, according to legend, the Chinese emperors had wonderful endurance, could do without sleep during long campaigns and did not lose vigor and internal balance. The wives of Chinese emperors numbered in the thousands - the rulers retained incredible potency until old age.

The first Chinese book on medicinal plants, in which lemongrass is given a place of honor, as well as descriptions of 900 medicinal plants, appeared 4,500 years ago. Many medicinal plants from this, as well as a number of other ancient Chinese pharmaceutical books that appeared after the first pharmacopoeia, became popular in other countries, thanks to the works of ancient Chinese scientists. These are lemongrass and ginseng, licorice root and motherwort, onion and garlic, cinnamon and camphor, ginger and skullcap.

Following the Chinese emperors, who introduced lemongrass berries 3 thousand years ago - from all over central China, the fruits were supposed to be delivered to the imperial palace - the whole world was convinced that it was impossible to find a second such plant that contains in all its parts a staggering amount of useful for human compounds, vitamins and minerals. In addition, lemongrass has one indisputable advantage even over ginseng, which in Chinese medicine has always been in first place in terms of its healing qualities: with optimal agricultural practices, the medicinal properties of cultivated lemongrass are absolutely no different from wild ones, which are already more than 25 million years old. Wild ginseng, unlike lemongrass, is much more useful than cultivated ginseng.

To one of the Chinese rulers, Cao Pi, emperor of the kingdom of Wei, who lived 18 centuries ago andwho patronized literature China): "With schizandra, you can go down to the underworld without soiling the toes of your shoes."

Schizandra - lemongrass - grew only in central China, and the need for it - as a well-known tonic and gastric remedy in the country - was increasing. And China even began to import lemongrass from abroad (schisandra grows in Korea, Japan, and in our Far East). Documents say that "through the port of Yingkou alone, 144,833 pounds of schisandra berries were imported into China in 1884 in connection with its use in Chinese medicine as a tonic."

Emperor Xuanzong of the Tang Dynasty, who ruled 13 centuries ago, is credited with lines in which the ruler admires schizandra - lemongrass - from the window. It is possible that the use of lemongrass helped the successful emperor to confidently rule the state.

Lemongrass has grown

picturesquely in the garden And even the light takes away:

Almost half of the window

Covered with bright green leaves; between them

The young brush in the window begins to blush.

Famous imperial baths with lemongrass fruits, cinnamon and red peony root or lemongrass fruits, peach flowers and Chinese rose, astragalus and ginseng roots are known.

The unique chemical composition of lemongrass

Schisandra chinensis is a unique medicine. This amazing plant owes, first of all, to its chemical composition.

Lemongrass berries contain sugars, organic acids, vitamins, minerals, pectins, as well as substances whose chemical composition has not yet been fully studied. The seeds contain tonic substances - schizandrin and schizandrol, vitamin E and oil, which consists of unsaturated fatty acids. There are absolutely no toxic substances in lemongrass. Dry berries of a medicinal plant retain vitamin C and a powerful tonic schizandrin in their composition. Lemongrass fruits and seeds are an excellent adaptogen, tonic and psychostimulant.

Saharalemongrass directly in finished form enter the bloodstream and are easily digested, without processing by digestive enzymes.

vitamins, which are found in lemongrass berries - this is vitamin C,PP, B1, E and beta-carotene.

Vitamin C (ascorbic acid)strengthensblood vessels, prevents atherosclerosis, improves immunity, prevents aging. It protects against infections and normalizes the activity of the endocrine system,and also provides elasticity to the skin and strengthens the mucous membranes.

Vitamin B1 (thiamine)contributes to the normal functioning of the nervous system, liver, heart, muscles, improves bowel function, improves skin, stimulates the brain, participates in fat, protein and water metabolism.

beta carotene(β-carotene), which is also found in the berry, protects against cancer, normalizes the functioning of the heart, strengthens the immune system, prevents premature aging of the body, that is, it is an antioxidant, has a great effect on vision, makes the skin soft and supple, heals mucous membranes.

PP (nicotinic acid, in Western countries - B3)participates in carbohydrate and protein metabolism, helps to reduce the levelcholesterol in the blood, lowers blood pressure, improves blood circulation, and also improves the functioning of the nervous system and brain, and has a beneficial effect on the functioning of the gastrointestinal tract.

Vitamin E (tocopherols and tocotrienols)important for the absorption of proteins and fats, for skin health, fights oxidation processes in the body, aging and cell death, has a good effect on the genitalglands, protects against carcinogens, has an anti-stress effect.

Tocopherol is number one of the antioxidants. Other antioxidants include vitamin C and beta-carotene.

Macro- and microelementsthat are in lemongrass are potassium, calcium, phosphorus, magnesium, copper, manganese, chromium, nickel, iodine, zinc, iron, selenium, cobalt, molybdenum, aluminum. Most minerals are found in lemongrass oil.

Potassiumensures the normal functioning of the heart and is responsible for removing fluid from the body, has a beneficial effect on the nervous system, participates in the synthesis of proteins, ATP (this acid is an energy accumulator in the cell) and glycogen (this substance is a storage of carbohydrates in liver and muscle cells). Potassium slows down the heart rate, helping in some cases to eliminate arrhythmias, and is involved in the transmission of signals from nerve endings.

Calciummakes strong bones and teeth, and muscles and internal organs - elastic. Calcium deficiency provokes the excitability of the nervous system and impaired blood clotting.

Phosphorustakes part in the production of proteins and the structure of cells. It has a beneficial effect on recovery, participates in the regulation of the nervous system.

Magnesiumstimulates intracellular reactions, helps to

assimilate other minerals, protects against the formation of malignant tumors. Magnesium deficiency provokes convulsions, numbness and tingling in the limbs, imbalance, fatigue, headaches, weather sensitivity, flashing "flies" before the eyes.

Copper- a necessary participant in the synthesis of red blood cells and collagen, which is responsible for skin elasticity, promotes the renewal of skin cells and the proper absorption of iron, participates in the processes of thermoregulation. Lack of copper provokes a violation of the pigmentation of hair and skin.

Manganeseimportant for oxidative processes and for the metabolism of fatty acids. It also controls cholesterol levels.

Chromiumcontrols the processing of carbohydrates, insulinexchange. Prolonged deficiency can lead to type 2 diabetes.

NickelIt is important as a stimulator of hematopoietic processes and an amplifier of oxidative processes in tissues, and is also of great importance for the functioning of the liver, pancreas, and pituitary gland.

Iodineregulates the functioning of the thyroid glandthe normal functioning of the endocrine system, kills microbes, and also strengthens the nervous system and nourishes the gray matter of the brain.

Zincparticipates in the production of insulin, in fat, protein and vitamin metabolism, in the synthesis of a number of hormones, increases male strength, and also stimulates general immunity, increases resistance to infections and counteracts nervous disorders.

Iron- an integral part of hemoglobin, iron affects the process of hematopoiesis and is necessary for the transport of oxygen by red blood cells, improves the functions of the muscular and nervous systems, helps with weakening of the body and fatigue.

Seleniumable to slow down the aging process and improve immunity, it belongs to the group of natural antioxidants. With a lack of selenium, the work of the heart may worsen and arrhythmias and shortness of breath may occur.

Cobaltis needed to activate the activity of a number of enzymes, to enhance the production of proteins, as well as to produce vitamin B12 and the formation of insulin.

Molybdenumstimulates fat and carbohydrate metabolism.

The lack of molybdenum causes problems with the digestion of food.

Aluminumnecessary for the growth and development of tissues - bone, connective and epithelial, for the processes of recovery andregeneration, regulation of the activity of enzymes and digestive glands.

organic acidslemongrass are represented by lemon, apple and wine. We need them mainly to normalize the work of the digestive organs: acids have an important positive effect on the metabolism of fats, reduce the level of cholesterol and total lipids in the blood (in addition to cholesterol, blood also contains other lipids). Acids help improve digestion by acting on gastric juice, and also reduce the risk of kidney stones.

Lemon acidremoves carcinogens and heavy metals from the body.

Apple acidcharacterized by anti-inflammatory

moisturizing and oxidizing properties and we need it forwell-established metabolism, good digestion and normal functioning of the excretory system.

Wine acidparticipates in metabolism, in respiratory processes, prevents the development of a number of microorganisms, helps the absorption of iron, improves the functioning of the digestive system.

Pectins- plant polysaccharides found in schisandra berries have excellent enterosorbent (binding and cleansing of harmful substances) properties, besides, they lower blood cholesterol levels, are a medicine for metabolic disorders, for malfunctions of the gastrointestinal tract and cardiovascular vascular system. If there is a normal amount of pectins in the body, harmful substances will not accumulate. In addition, pectin substances improve peripheral blood circulation and promote the excretion of radionuclides, pesticides, heavy metal ions from the body.

Lemongrass seeds contain tonic substances - schizandrin and schizandrol, vitamin tocopherol, fatty acids and essential oils.

Lemongrass oil is an excellent tonic, immunity booster, a treasure trove of macronutrients and vitamins.

Fatty acids are represented

mainly by linoleic, linolenic and oleic.

Fatty acidis a building material for fats in our body. The biological value of unsaturated fats is higher, since their effect on fat metabolism in the body is more favorable.

Linoleic and linolenic acidsbelong to the group of polyunsaturated fatty acids Omega-6. Both acids help reduce blood cholesterol levels, are involved in the synthesis of sex hormones and adrenal hormones (regulating blood pressure, for example); activate the function of the peripheral and central nervous system, reduce the content of excess cholesterol in the blood, increase immunity.

Oleic acidis a fatty monounsaturated acid belonging to the group of omega-9 acids. It is part of the fats involved in the construction of cell membranes. This acid determines the composition of building fats. If oleic acid is replaced by any other, the permeability of cell membranes changes.

Due to the oleic composition, fats are resistant to oxidation with a moderate presence of antioxidant substances (antioxidants) in the body.

Oleic acid is synthesized in the human liver, but its intake with food is also necessary for the formation of a fat depot on this basis. Oleic acid actively counteracts the development of osteoporosis (that is, leaching of calcium from the bones), reduces the risk of atherosclerosis (prevents the deposition of cholesterol plaques on the walls of blood vessels), and has a beneficial effect on the function of the gastrointestinal tract, on the functioning of the liver and gallbladder.

In all parts of lemongrass, without exception, there is an essential oil - itvery actively used in perfumery and is distinguished by an exquisitely spicy lemon scent.

The essential oil contained in the bark of the plant has the appearance of a mobile transparent golden liquid with a lemon scent.

The most important and unique

substances contained in lemongrass are lignans, which have a very wide range of biological activity. They are found in leaves, berries, plant bark and rhizomes. Many scientists believe that it is thanks to lignans that lemongrass has antitumor, antifungal,tonic, antimicrobial and anti-inflammatory action, and is also a powerful antioxidant.

Antioxidants are substances that prevent oxidation processes in the body. Oxidation products (otherwise called "free radicals"), like rust, damage cell membranes, and cells lose their protective properties. The accumulation of free radicals is a sign of body aging. If the body is saturated with antioxidants, much less oxidation products accumulate, and the metabolism normalizes. Antioxidants (free radical scavengers) are a good way to rejuvenate our body.

Lemongrass is a terrific adaptogen as lignans stimulate the central nervous system.

Adaptogens have a unique property to enhance the resistance of a living organism in difficult or extreme conditions. In folk medicine, they have been used for many centuries as prophylactic agents. If adaptogens are used constantly, health improves, resistance to diseases increases.

Lignans belong to the group of antioxidants and improve liver function. But still, their main quality is a tonic effect on the body. The lignans schizadrin and schizandrol have an exciting effect on the nervous system, increasing efficiency and stimulating the work of the heart, blood vessels, respiratory and central nervous system. The amazing substance schizandrin has a particularly strong effect.

The most effective substances of lemongrassowing to which it - as a healing agent - is in oriental medicine in second place after ginseng and has a unique spectrum of effects - these are schizandrin, schizandrol, essential oils, sugars, citric and malic acids.

It is not surprising that with such an unprecedented composition, lemongrass serves as a concentrated elixir of healing, rejuvenation, and tenfold strength!

The main healing secrets of lemongrass

For the first time, lemongrass as a healing agent that perfectly relieves fatigue and restores strength, tones and stimulates the body, was mentioned in a Chinese treatise about two and a half thousand years ago. For centuries, it has been actively used in Chinese, Japanese, Korean, and then in Russian folk medicine.

Later, in the twentieth century, scientists figured out why this happens by studying the chemical composition of the plant. Studies have been conducted on the effects of lemongrass during sports, long transitions, prolonged mental and physical work, and in a number of serious diseases. It turned out that a number of amazing qualities should be added to the tonic and restorative properties of lemongrass.

The ancient Chinese sages wrote about the healing power of lemongrass as follows: “Schisandra strengthens muscles, warms the insides. Two hours after taking the medicine, hearing and vision become more acute, fatigue disappears, and metabolism improves.

Lemongrass has been proven to:

improves the body's resistance to various diseases; enhances metabolism and immunity, rejuvenates body cells; increases defenses in general;

is an adaptogen: it accelerates the body's adaptation to a sharp change in external factors;

improves the general condition of the body, appetite, sleep;

increases mental and physical abilities; increases efficiency with strong physical stress, physical and mental fatigue, drowsiness, depressive states;

neededwith a breakdown due to infectious diseases;

burns unnecessary fats and improves carbohydrate metabolism;

enhances reflexes;

stimulates the heart and blood vessels; fights atherosclerosis, helps with anemia;

regulates blood circulation;

increases blood pressure;

decreases heart rate by increasing

increases the content of hemoglobin in the blood;

increases the body's resistance to oxygen starvation;

excites the respiratory center;

necessary in the treatment of tuberculosis, bronchitis, bronchial asthma,pneumonia;

a drop of lemongrass oil applied to the sinuses of the nose,

improves motor and secretory functions of the gastrointestinal tractpath;

helps with gastritis with high

acidity, as well as withlow acidity of gastric juice; with chronic gastritis;

has a beneficial effect on the functions of the liver and gallbladder, as well as the kidneys;

reduces the amount of sugar in the blood, therefore it is indicated for diabetes mellitus;

improves the work of the genitourinary sphere; helps with sexual weakness;

improves night vision;

stimulates labor activity;

copes well with scurvy - not only fruits are a powerful antiscorbutic agent, but also an infusion of leaves or bark of magnolia vine;

stimulates sexual activity;

relieves stress and hangover syndrome;

stabilizes sleep;

helps with skin diseases; accelerates its regeneration;

promotes healing of wounds, including trophic ulcers;

used in the complex treatment of oncological diseases. Lemongrass is a perfect stimulant in its action. In people,

who are generally healthy, this plant prevents the feeling of fatigue (which is why it should be used at the first sign offatigue), enhances resistance to extreme factors, for example, it will help to successfully acclimatize during climate change.

fruit of five flavors maintains excellent health, increases efficiency, thus helping to cope with enormouspressures of modern life. Lemongrass will remove lethargy and harmonize mood, increase excitation in the cerebral cortex and reflex activity of the central nervous system. The result is a faster and more efficient assimilation of any new information. In addition, the cardiovascular and respiratory systems will begin to work much better.

Lemongrass is not effective in organic diseases of the heart and blood vessels, such as heart disease, myocardial dystrophy, cardiosclerosis, angina pectoris.

Scientists tested lemongrass and phenamine on healthy people aged 18–27 years. It turned out that under the influence of several schisandra berries, the condition of the subjects improved significantly, there was a surge of vivacity, strength, increased motor activity and efficiency, night vision increased, the desire to sleep disappeared, and muscle strength increased. And all this without any side effects. Phenamine administration gave similar results. But after a few hours and the next day after taking phenamine, fatigue, general weakness, nausea, headache and palpitations occurred, which was not the case with lemongrass. The absence of side effects makes it possible to attribute lemongrass to an unprecedentedly valuable tonic and stimulant.

Lemongrass will help to adapt to any stress, physicaland mental, will increase immunity and will be a wonderful prevention of influenza and acute respiratory diseases, since it significantly increases the body's defenses.

Eating lemongrass during the flu season reduces the risk of getting sick by about five times.

Both healthy people and those who suffer from low blood pressure, asthenic syndrome, and vegetative-vascular dystonia of the hypotonic type can use Schizandra preparations to increase tone.

An amazing stimulating refreshing effect is especially noticeable during hard work, which requires concentration, integrity of perception or precise coordination of movements and is associated with high psychophysiological costs. Lemongrass has a positive effect on the senses, especially on the visual system: it increases visual acuity and improves eye adaptation to darkness.

At the same time, lemongrass works in such a way that its tonic effect does not deplete the nervous system.

Studies by scientists have shown that during heavy physical exertion (pulling up on the arms), people who had previously taken a course of lemongrass tincture almost completely retained their physical strength, while in the rest of the subjects, physical strength sharply decreased after exercise. And observations that were made in the troops at especially high levels of fatigue proved that lemongrass prevents the development of fatigue.

Lemongrass should be used by people who have a breakdown due to infectious diseases, reduced tone of the heart system, low blood pressure, low efficiency,asthenic syndrome, depression, poor digestion, weakness of smooth and skeletal muscles, sexual dysfunction against the background of neurasthenia.

Lemongrass is highly effective for gastritis - it quickly normalizes the composition of gastric juice. It turns out that even a single dose of 2 g of seed powder increases low acidity and reduces high acidity.

With cholecystitis and biliary dyskinesia, lemongrass will return both the liver and gallbladder to normal.

Dermatologists actively use the medicinal properties of lemongrass in such diseases as alopecia, vitiligo, vasculitis, allergic dermatosis, lichen planus, viral and blistering dermatitis.

A healthy skin Lemongrasswill make you younger and more beautiful, being a very good home beautician.

Lemongrass - on the advice of a doctor - it is better to take regularly, and not one-time. The maximum effect comes in half a month. If you take lemongrass along with vitamins, the effect will increase. To avoid allergic reactions, you need to check exactly how this or that Schizandra preparation works for you: take a very small dose 20 minutes before a meal or a few hours after a meal. The reaction can be felt in about half an hour.

The usual scheme for taking lemongrass is as follows: the medicine (tincture, infusion, decoction, etc.) is consumed on an empty stomach or 4 hours after a meal. The action of Schisandra manifests itself in half an hour and lasts up to six hours. Currently, a pharmacy tincture is made from the fruits and seeds of lemongrass in 96% alcohol.

In the Far East, the juice of lemongrass berries is used as a food acid, jelly, fruit drinks, various drinks are prepared, and the bark of the stems, which smells like lemon, is added to tea.

Interesting observations about the effect of lemongrass on vision were made at the Helmholtz Institute. In healthy people, the sensitivity of vision was measured before consuming lemongrass every 5 minutes for an hour. When the night vision indicators stabilized, the subject was given 1.6 g of lemongrass powder, and then the sensitivity of vision was measured again within an hour or two. Night vision acuity improved significantly! For an adultthe optimal dose that enhances night vision is no more than 1.5-2 g of lemongrass seeds.

The main working substances of lemongrass are physiological antagonists of sleeping pills and drugs that depress the central nervous system. And the action of psychostimulants and analeptics (including caffeine, camphor and phenamine) magnolia vine, on the contrary, enhances.

Lemongrass as a tonic and stimulating drug should be taken only after a medical examination and under periodic medical supervision. After 18-19 hours, lemongrass should not be consumed, otherwise you will have a sleepless night.

Contraindications to the use of

Contraindicationsfor lemongrass:

hypertension;

increased intracranial pressure;

increased nervous excitability;

insomnia;

violations of cardiac activity;

acute infectious diseases;

stomach ulcer;

chronic liver diseases;

epilepsy;

hypersensitivity to the components of the drug;

pregnancy and lactation;

Schisandra should not be taken by children under 12 years of age.

Adverse reactionsthat can be observed when using lemongrass:

tachycardia;

allergic reactions;

sleep disorders;

headache;

increase in blood pressure.

According to research by doctors, in 4% of people, lemongrass can cause lethargy and depression of the nervous system.

In case of an overdose, overexcitation of the nervous and cardiovascular systems is possible.

And one more nuance - in the spring,during the period of juice saturation, it is not recommended to use lemongrass vine (for infusions, teas, decoctions) - during this period the plant has very strong activity, the heart and blood vessels may react too violently.

Lemongrass is a very powerful remedy, so before you start taking lemongrass in any form, you should consult a doctor.

Chapter 2 The Berry That Gives

You will recognize five taste sensations when you find a thin liana

With a lemon scent of bark and leaves. Bunch of red berries

if you can take it off -

It will add strength to you on a long journey, And you will surprise yourself with the sparkle of your eyes When you look into the mirror of the stream.

Alexander Buzni

If lemongrass grows in your country house, then you need to collect its berries for medicinal purposes in September, when they have a tart taste and cause a characteristic burning sensation in your mouth.

Important: when collecting or processing lemongrass berriesit is strictly forbidden to use easily oxidized dishes - this can lead to poisoning.

To increase physical and mental activity and endurance

When using lemongrass preparations to increase mental and physical performance, a doctor's recommendation is required.

Tincture of berries and leaves of lemongrass to increase efficiency

Tinctureworks great as a stimulant of the body, increases strength, protects against colds, lethargy, dystonia, beriberi. Existstwo common methods of making tinctures: from the lemongrass fruit and from the plant itself. You can use both 70% and 96% alcohol.

You need to take 1 part of lemongrass fruits (both ripe and dried) and 5 parts of alcohol of 70% concentration, pour lemongrass fruits into a dark glass dish and pour alcohol. Insist in a dark cool place for 10 days, periodically shaking the contents. Then the tincture is filtered and stored in a dark glass sealed container in a cool place protected from bright light. Usual way of application: 2 times a day (preferably in the morning and in the afternoon) 20-30 drops 20-30 minutes before meals. The duration of the course is 1 month.

You need to take 1 part of the chopped plant (washed leaves, shoots) to 3 parts of 70% alcohol. In a dark glass bowl, mix alcohol and stems and leaves. Insist in a dark and cool place for 8-10 days. Then strain. The tincture from the plant must be taken either on an empty stomach or 4 hours after eating 2-3 times a day, 20-30 drops each. The course is the same: 3-4 weeks.

Lemongrass seed tincture

It restores strength, stimulates mental and physical activity, strengthens the body as a whole, is a vitamin complex that improves the functioning of the nervous and immune systems. Alsoit is recommended to use the tincture with an increase in the acidity of the stomach, hypotension, drowsiness, decreased attention, during the period of physical and mental adaptation, with deterioration of various sensitivities (hearing, vision, etc.).

50 g lemongrass seeds

0.5 l vodka

Rinse the lemongrass seeds well to remove the remnants of the berry. Then they are thoroughly crushed and pour vodka. Place in a dark place for 14 days. The finished tincture is used 25 drops up to 3 times a day.

To enhance physical and mental activity, you can prepare an infusion of lemongrass berries. Both fresh and dried berries are suitable. Dried fruits of lemongrass must be brewed as tea and drunk to raise the tone of the body and relieve fatigue, as well as against scurvy. How to dry? Slightly dried lemongrass berries should be put on a baking sheet in one layer and put in the oven, preheated to 60 C. You need to dry in 3-4 doses for several days.

Infusion of lemongrass berries

15 g lemongrass fruits

300 ml boiling water

Pour boiling water over chopped berries, heat over low heat, without boiling, for 15 minutes. Take 1 tablespoon 2-3 times a day, but no later than 5 hours before bedtime.

For the winter, lemongrass can be prepared in the form of fresh berries in sugar. A very effective tool for always being in good working shape.

Fresh berries in sugar

The berries are slightly dried, covered with sugar in a ratio of 1: 2, mixed, placed in glass jars, covered with lids or paper and stored in a cool place. Used as an additive to tea.

Tea or an infusion of lemongrass leaves and shoots, both fresh and dried, will increase your strength. Leaves, stems, bark of lemongrass act on the body more gently than berries and preparations from berries, since they contain less tonic substances than fruits. Infusion and tea relieves depression well.

In August, it is advisable to prepare the leaves and young (one- and two-year-old) shoots, chop them, lay them out in a thin layer on paper and dry in a shaded place that is well ventilated. Then store in a dark cool place. Can be stored in cloth bags.

Tea from leaves and shootslemongrass

Tea is brewed at the rate of 1 teaspoon of crushed leaves orlemongrass shoots (fresh or dry) to 1 cup boiling water. To brew or infuse any parts of lemongrass (as well as any other medicinal plant), you need glass, enameled or stainless steel dishes with a tight-fitting lid. It is recommended to filter decoctions or infusions through a tea - faience or silver - strainer. You can filter decoctions and infusions through 2-4 layers of gauze.

To enhance mental and physical performance, lemongrass oil is perfect, which contains a huge amount of biologically active substances. Experts say that it enhances performance by two to three times! In addition, this oil has an anti-inflammatory effect, improves the functioning of the gastrointestinal tract and is distinguished by anti-cancer activity. The oil is also indicated for overwork, in extreme situations (hypothermia, overheating, radiation), after infectious and prolonged illnesses. It will help students and schoolchildren - their ability to memorize and assimilate new material will increase significantly. Lemongrass oil improves night vision. It is used by athletes, including the Russian Olympic football and hockey teams (limongrass oil is not doping). Lemongrass oil is sold in pharmacies.

lemongrass oil

You need to take lemongrass oil 1 capsule of 0.1 g before meals.Course - 10 days. Then take a break for 20 days and repeat the course 1 or 2 times. Such techniques are shown in autumn and spring. With severe fatigue, a single dose of 3-4 capsules is allowed. Oil should not be taken after 6 pm. Contraindications for taking are the same as for any lemongrass preparations. Before taking the oil, you should consult your doctor.

To increase mental and physical activity and endurance, as well as to restore strength, you can take the powderfrom lemongrass seeds. The powder reduces fatigue during heavy physical exertion. Great for the sick and the healthy! In particular, when working on a night shift, when working with large overloads. After taking the powder, about half an hour later, an increase in strength begins, mood improves, and working capacity increases - both physical and mental. The feeling of cheerfulness can last up to 8 hours. The powder is not addictive.

Lemongrass seed powder

You need to take 1-3 g of lemongrass seed powder per day. The course of admission for medicinal purposes is 3 weeks.

Single doses of lemongrass in any form are ineffective. The usual course is from three weeks to one month. The peak of exposure to lemongrass preparations falls on the 15-20th day of the course.

Remarkably multiplies and restores strength natural juice from lemongrass berries.

Natural juice from lemongrass berries

Method 1.Wash the berries, squeeze the juice in a juicer. Pour the finished juice into clean jars and sterilize, seal tightly. Store in a cold place. For use, 1 teaspoon of lemongrass juice is diluted in 200 ml of hot water. Juice is added to tea or coffee 1-1.5 teaspoons 2 times a day with a decrease in tone and overwork.

Method 2.Squeeze the washed

berries in a juicer. Pour the remaining pomace with hot water 1:1 and squeeze the juice again. Mix the juice of the first and second extractions, strain, pour into an enamel pan, heat to 95 ° C and pour into jars while hot. Sterilize jars, seal tightly. Store in a cold place.

After making juice from lemongrass fruits, we still have squeezes. From these pressings you can make wine that will not only give strength to perform any work, increase tone, but also quench your thirst.

Tonic lemongrass wine

A lot of pulp remains in the squeezes, seeds must be removed from it, then the squeezes must be poured with cold water and kept for 2–3 days to extract dyes and vitamins. Drain the must and add sugar. Due to the high acidity, the wort must be well diluted with water. If this is not done, then excess acid will block fermentation ahead of time. But even very weak lemongrass wine does not spoil for a long time. Its main use is to dilute the wine twice with good water (preferably from a well) and drink it instead of water in the summer, at the very hot time.

Lemongrass compote

This compote raises efficiency and relieves fatigue.

Prepare syrup from 5 liters of water and 2.5 kg of sugar. Place well-washed fresh lemongrass fruits in sterilized jars and carefully pour over hot syrup. Then sterilize for 5 minutes. After the jars have cooled, place them in a cool place.

lemongrass jam

Jam will give strength, strengthen the body, remove hypotension.

600 ml water

1.25 kg sugar

1 kg lemongrass berries

Boil the syrup, pour it with well-washed lemongrass fruits. Let stand for an hour and a half, then put on fire and boil for 5 minutes. Then cool and arrange in jars. Store in a cool place.

Lemongrass and Dandelion Leaf Tea

1-2 teaspoons crushed dandelion leaves and roots

1 tablespoon chopped lemongrass leaves

250 g cold water

I pour dandelion and lemongrass with water, boil for one minute, and filter after 10 minutes. I drink three times a day.

Lemongrass, Dandelion, Nettle and Green Tea Balm

This balm - due to its healing composition - perfectly tones the body, rejuvenates it and cleanses the blood.

1 tablespoon dry lemongrass leaves

3 tablespoons dandelion root

4 tablespoons nettle leaves

5 tablespoons green tea

1 cup hotwater

Prepare a mixture of dried and crushed ingredients: lemongrass leaves, dandelion root, green tea, nettle leaves. Mix everything well. Brew hot water 2 teaspoons of the resulting mixture. Leave for 15 minutes, then strain. Drink 2-3 times a day for 1/3 cup.

Dandelion along with nettle and lemongrass,Yes, even with green tea, it increases vitality tenfold and is the prevention of many diseases.

All parts of dandelion are healing and help to improve the body, normalize metabolism. The most valuable juice is obtained from the leaves and roots. Dandelion heals many ailments, increases hemoglobin, cleanses the blood and lymph, heals nerves, calms, induces sound sleep, increases appetite, and reduces weight.

Nettle is a vitamin, an immunocorrector, and an antiseptic! Herb from almost all diseases, it restores metabolic processes for years to come, it is necessary if the work of the liver, gallbladder, gastrointestinal tract is disrupted, if joints hurt, if blood sugar is elevated, and immunity is lowered, if there are cardiovascular diseases , allergies, skin diseases. Nettle removes excess cholesterol, toxins, toxins, increases hemoglobin, strengthens cartilage, renews mucous membranes, stimulates the work of all internal organs, alleviates stress, relieves inflammation, and normalizes acid-base balance.

Contraindicationsto the use of nettle in any form: acute heart and kidney failure, pregnancy, increased blood clotting, thrombophlebitis, gastritis, ulcers, hypertension, atherosclerosis.

Nettle Lemon Tea

2 heaping teaspoons minced nettle leaves and rhizomes

2 teaspoons chopped dried lemongrass leaves

1/4 liter boiling water

I make tea like this: pour boiling water over nettles and lemongrass, boil for 5 minutes and filter. I drink warm, in small sips, 1 cup in the morning and in the evening for one to two months.

Lemongrass, rosehip, raisins, nettle

I dry nettles in the summer, I also harvest rose hipssummer, lemongrass

at the beginning of autumn. I

make raisins from my own grapes. But you can also buy.

All of the above components, brought together, give a lot of strength, heal the body and increase immunity. Nettle also cleanses the blood.

2 tablespoons crushed dried lemongrass

3 tablespoons crushed dried rose hips

1 tablespoon raisins

3 tablespoons dried minced nettle leaves

500 ml boiling water

I pour 1 tablespoon of the mixture with 500 ml of boiling water, boil over low heat for 10 minutes, then insist in a dark, warm place for 4 hours. I filter and drink 1/2 cup 3-4 times a day half an hour before meals.

The value of wild rose lies in the exceptionally high content of ascorbic acid (vitamin C). Rose hips are rich in antioxidants and have antibacterial properties. In folk medicine, it is used as a multivitamin remedy, as well as an adjuvant in the treatment of diseases of the liver, kidneys, bladder, heart and blood vessels. Rosehip tea has a mild diuretic property that does not require a replacement intake of potassium. Important: fresh fruits can be irritating to the gastrointestinal tract.

Raisins are not only an

immunostimulant, but also a tonic for the heart and blood vessels, for the nervous system. Raisins contain many antioxidants.

Lemongrass, nettle, yarrow and dandelion

1 part crushed lemongrass

1 part minced nettle leaves

1 part crushed yarrow flowers

1 part chopped dandelion root

1.5 cups boiling water

Brew a tablespoon of the mixture with boiling water, leave for 3 hours,strain.

Drink a day in 3-4 doses 20 minutes before meals. Course - 8 weeks.

Yarrow has a wonderfulgeneral strengthening action. It contains a lot of vitamin C, it strengthens the walls of blood vessels well. In addition, this plant has a great effect on the gastrointestinal tract, relieves pain in gastritis, is indicated for liver diseases, is used for bronchopulmonary diseases asantibacterial, expectorant, anti-inflammatory agent.

Lemongrass, wild rose, tea kopeechnik

1 part crushed lemongrass

1 part crushed rose hips

1 part chopped chamomile herb

1.5 cups boiling water

Tablespoon of the mixture brew with boiling water, leave for 2 hours

Kopeck tea (red root) - excellentgeneral tonic and stimulant, it treats diseases of the urogenital area, anemia.

Lemongrass, rosehip, nettle and lingonberry

Such tea will not only add mental and physical activity, but also help with beriberi.

1 teaspoon crushed lemongrass

3 tablespoons crushed rose hips

2 tablespoons cranberries

3 tablespoons minced nettle leaves

250 ml boiling water

Mix all the ingredients and pour 4 tablespoons of the mixture with boiling water. Infuse for at least 3 hours, drink in the morning and in the afternoon 30 minutes before meals. Well

one month.

Lingonberry is a multivitamin remedy, it has a vasoconstrictive, anti-sclerotic, choleretic, diuretic and disinfectant effect. Lingonberry improves metabolism, is useful for the prevention of colds, and has the ability to quickly remove toxins. Important: you can not eat a lot of lingonberries with increasedacidity of gastric juice, cholecystitis. Cowberry leaves and juice lower blood pressure, so lingonberries should be used with caution in case of hypotension.

Lemongrass and apple juice

1 kg fruitlemongrass

1.5 kg sugar

0.5 cup apple juice

Rinse the berries, scald with boiling water, rub through a sieve, add sugar and apple juice, cook until tender. Store in a cool place.

Lemongrass with dodder and mummy with a breakdown for the elderly Oriental medicine recommends this infusion for the elderly with

a decline in strength, but it can also be used by those who are younger - to enhance mental and physical endurance and activity.

1 part minced lemongrass fruits and seeds

1 part crushed dodder fruit and seeds

1 cup boiling water

a piece of mummy

You need to take 2 teaspoons of a mixture of equal parts of crushed fruits and seeds of lemongrass and dodder, pour boiling water and add a piece of mummy the size of a match head. Cover the glass with a towel and leave for 30 minutes. Then strain. Take 2 times in the morning. After 15 hours, it is better not to take the infusion - there may be insomnia. The course of admission is 20 days, then a break for 20 days and repetition of treatment.

To increase efficiency, increase mental and physical endurance, almost all the recipes that are given in the same chapter in the sections "To increase immunity" and "To improve metabolism" are suitable.

To improve immunity

When using lemongrass preparations to increase immunity, a doctor's recommendation is required.

Traditional medicine in particular and medicine in general have in their arsenal many ways to increase immunity with the help of lemongrass. I have used many of the recipes listed here. There are more complicated recipes, there are simpler ones, but all of them work to strengthen the immune system.

To increase immunity, you can drink pharmacy tincture of lemongrass berries 20-40 drops 2 times a day or take fruit powder

0.5 g in the morning and evening, but no later than 4 hours before bedtime. All this is taken on an empty stomach or 4 hours after a meal.

You can make alcohol tincture of lemongrass at home. Alcohol tincture of lemongrass

This tincture is sold in pharmacies, but you can make it at home. It is used as a vitamin, tonic, tonic that improves the functioning of the nervous and immune systems, it is especially good for asthenia and nervous breakdown.

20 g ripeor dry lemongrass

100 ml 70% alcohol

Grind lemongrass berries, pour

into a dark glass bottle, pour alcohol, close tightly and infuse for 10 days at room temperature in a dark place. The bottle must be shaken from time to time. After that, strain the tincture, squeeze the berries and leave for another two days, then strain again. Now the tincture should become transparent. Take 20-30 drops 2 times a day, morning and afternoon 30 minutes before meals. The course of treatment is from 20 to 35 days.

To raise immunity, lemongrass fruits can simply be chewed (no more than 5 berries per day, the course is 1 month), brew tea from them (10 g of dry crushed fruits per 0.5 l of boiling water). And you can prepare a wonderful tonic decoction: boil 1 tablespoon of fruits in a glass of water in an enamel bowl for 10 minutes, leave for a day, then strain and add sugar to taste.

Stimulating infusion

A wonderful tool for increasing efficiency, improving immunity, eliminating stress and depression, with chronic fatigue, with various overloads.

1 tablespoon fresh or dried lemongrass

1 cup boiling water

Berries insist in a thermos for 2 hours, strain and take 2 tablespoons before meals 4 times a day.

A decoction of dried lemongrass

1 tablespoon dry lemongrass

1 glass of water

Boil the fruits in an enamel bowl for 10 minutes, then let it brew for 24 hours, strain and add sugar to taste.

Berries and lemongrass juicecan be added to tea: 3-5 berries or 1 teaspoon per glass of tea. But it's better not to do it every day.

Tonic tea

Grind lemongrass leaves or branches, pour boiling water over, insist like regular tea. This tonic tea has a pleasant taste. The berries, leaves and bark of lemongrass are used as an antiscorbutic.

Lemongrass leaves or branches tea is an excellent substitute for natural tea. It has a beautiful golden color, perfectly relieves fatigue, soothes, adds strength, refreshes in the heat, has a lemon scent.

Leaves and stems have a milder effect than lemongrass berries, as they contain less tonic substances.

Water infusion of leaves and infusions of lemongrass bark have long been used by folk medicine as an excellent vitamin and antiscorbutic remedy.

Vitamin juice from freshfruits

You can make juice from fresh lemongrass fruits, which can significantly improve immunity. Freshly picked fruits are washed, squeezed in a juicer and immediately sterilized in small bottles. One teaspoon of this juice is enough to give the tea a great health and pleasant taste.

Natural fresh juice is stored in the refrigerator for a long time without losing its beneficial properties. It can be diluted with water and get a tonic and refreshing drink with lemon flavor.

Juice from dried lemongrass

If you did not have time to squeeze the juice from fresh berries, you can also make it from dried ones.

1 kg drylemongrass fruits

1.5 liters of water

Place the berries in an enamel pan, pour water, close the lid and boil for 10 minutes, then leave for 10-12 hours, strain, add sugar to taste, heat until sugar dissolves, bottle. In a well-closed glass container, juice can be stored in the refrigerator for a long time.

According to scientists, any person develops age-related immunodeficiency with age, since the thymus (thymus gland), which is the central organ of the immune system, is approximately

At the age of 40, it already has very low activity, and life expectancy, experts believe, is directly related to the so-called thymic activity. Lemongrass - in any form - has the ability to stimulate thymic activity, increasing life expectancy.

Infusion of lemongrass shoots

Annual shoots are crushed, put in a liter jar and poured with vodka. After 3 weeks, a viscous liquid resembling jelly is obtained. Take the infusion as follows: a teaspoon per glass of tea. Drink usually in the morning. It is very useful for colds and in winter as a prevention of acute respiratory infections.

Stimulating wine

Healing wine can be made from lemongrass. The fruits of lemongrass are crushed, 3 parts of water are added, sugar by weight of the fruit (1: 1).

Lemongrass compote

Prepared lemongrass fruits pour 40% sugarsyrup or boiled water and pasteurize for 15 minutes. Then clog.

Lemongrass mashed with sugar

Add sugar (60-65%) to mashed fruits (35-40%), mix thoroughly to evenly distribute sugar, heat to 70 C and package in hot sterilized glass jars. Roll up.

lemongrass jam

1 kg fruitlemongrass

1.5 kg sugar

Pass the sorted and washed fruits through a stainless steel sieve. Add sugar to the puree and cook, stirring, with a slight boil until tender. Pack the jam in hot sterilized jars, roll up.

Apple-lemon juice

Add lemongrass (20%) and sugar (25%) to apple juice (55%).

%). To stir thoroughly. Heat the mixture, stirring constantly, until the sugar dissolves, bring to a boil, boil for 3-4 minutes and immediately pour into hot sterilized jars. Roll up.

Lemongrass, raisinand wild rose

Drinking this decoction is a very simple way to boost immunity. In addition, the decoction has anti-inflammatory and blood-purifying effects. The last property is important for the skin - it will look younger. This decoction can be drunk all autumn, winter and spring in monthly courses, then take a break for a month. Its components are always available to us. They are easy to stock up from the summer.

1 tablespoon crushed dried lemongrass

3 tablespoons crushed dry rose hips

1 tablespoon raisins

3 tablespoons crushed dried grape leaves

2.5 cups boiling water

Pour boiling water over the prepared mixture, cook on low heat for 10 minutes, then insist in a dark, warm place for 4 hours. Strain and drink 1/2 cup 3-4 times a day.

Infusion of lemongrass and rose hips

3 tablespoons rose hips

2 tablespoons chopped lemongrass stems or leaves

0.5 l boiling water

Brew in a thermos at night and drink 2-3 times a day as tea. Blueberry lemon juice

To blueberry juice (50%) add lemongrass (20%) and sugar (30

%). Bring the mixture to a boil, stirring constantly, boil for 3-5 minutes and immediately pour into hot sterilized jars. Roll up.

Blueberry strengthens blood vessels, normalizes the functioning of the intestines and pancreas, improves metabolismsubstances, different

Lemongrass and black elderberry

This infusion will not only boost immunity, but also help with colds.

1 teaspoon crushed lemongrass

1 tablespoon dried elderberry flowers

1 cup boiling water

Pour lemongrass and elderberry with boiling water, leave for 20 minutes, strain. Infusion take 1/4 cup (preferably with honey) 3 times a day 15 minutes before meals.

Black elder among many peoples is known as a sacred plant - due to its healing properties. The plant improves immunity, improves metabolism, normalizes the functioning of the gastrointestinal tract, is useful in diabetes mellitus, has a diuretic, diaphoretic, antipyretic, anti-inflammatory and disinfectant effect. Decoctions and infusions of black elderberry help with influenza, respiratory diseases, bronchitis, pneumonia, diseases of the bladder and kidneys.

Herbal collection: lemongrass, nettle, sage

Such a drink will boost immunity and help not get sick during the flu season and acute respiratory infections.

3 partsnettle leaf

3 parts lemongrass shoots

1 part sage herb

1 cup boiling water

1 teaspoonhoney

Boiling water is poured into a thermos 1 teaspoon of crushed collection, insist 1-2 hours and drink after breakfast, adding honey.

Sage is rich in antioxidants and vitamins,has antimicrobial andanti-inflammatory effect, beneficial effect on the gastrointestinal tract, stimulates mental activity. In the old days, tea was brewed from it “for inspiration”. Sage helps with any problems with the throat, is indicated for inflammation of the genitourinary system, with cholecystitis, colitis, mild forms of diabetes, pulmonary tuberculosis, and is part of chest collections.

The plant is contraindicated during pregnancy, as well as in acute nephritis.

Tea with lemongrass, raspberries and currants

5 g drylemongrass berries

5 g dried raspberries

5 g dry blackcurrants

Brew berries like tea and drink 3 times a day half an hour before meals.

Raspberries are indispensable for colds, indicated for anemia, problems with the gastrointestinal tract, atherosclerosis, kidney disease, hypertension. It has antipyretic, hemostatic and antitoxic properties, it improves appetite, helps the skin to be healthy. Raspberries contain copper, which is part of many antidepressants. Therefore, raspberry helps with great nervous stress.

Blackcurrant is a wonderful immune stimulant. Helps eliminate problems with the cardiovascular system, prevents the weakening of intellectual abilities in the elderly, is indicated for diseases of the kidneys, liver and respiratory tract, with atherosclerosis, has a restorative, disinfectant and anti-inflammatory effect, helps with hypertension, anemia, gastritis, gastric and duodenal ulcers, bleeding gums. Strong antiseptic.

Honey-lemon tincture

This tincture is an excellent immunostimulant.

10 bunches of berries

1 liter of vodka

2 tablespoons honey

Lemongrass berry tincture tastes like cranberry liqueur. It is necessary to fill the brushes of lemongrass berries with vodka, put in a dark place, and after a month add honey. Take 30 drops 2 times a day, morning and afternoon 30 minutes before meals. The course is up to 35 days.

Before the berries ripen, you can make tinctures from the stems and leaves of lemongrass with the addition of rose hips.

Lemongrass and rosehipwith honey

Such a tool gives a lot of strength, stimulates the immune system, improves tone and mood.

3 stalks of lemongrass with leaves

10 rose hips

2 tablespoons honey

0.5 l vodka

Finely chop three stems about half a meter long with leaves with scissors, add rose hips cut with a knife. Pour vodka, put in a dark place, after a month add honey. The tincture is ready to use. It is more dense, oily, and tastes softer than lemongrass berry tincture. They can be mixed, or you can take separate courses. Take 30 drops 2 times a day, morning and afternoon 30 minutes before meals. The course is up to 35 days.

Rosehip - vitamin C concentrate. Rosehiprich in antioxidants has antibacterial properties. In folk medicine, it is used as a multivitamin remedy, as well as an adjuvant in the treatment of diseases of the liver, kidneys, bladder, heart and blood vessels.

To increase immunity, almost all the recipes that are given in the same chapter in the sections "To increase mental and physical

endurance" and "To activate metabolism" are suitable.

To activate metabolism

When using drugslemongrass to activate the metabolism, a doctor's recommendation is required.

Metabolism is regulated by two systems: the endocrine and central nervous systems. And if these balance controllers in the body find something wrong with our metabolic processes, they turn on SOS signals - either by a jump in pressure, or by pain in the joints or in the stomach. Alarm signals can be very different and unexpected - weight gain, nervous irritability, increased susceptibility to colds. The body fails here and there, we treat individual diseases, but it is the metabolism that needs to be treated. Then some diseases will go away. If we do not deal with the root cause, that is, metabolic processes, we risk earning chronic diseases - such as diabetes, thyroid disease, gout, obesity.

Between the metabolic processes in the human body and the microelements that make up the structure of plants, a subtle and strong agreement has long been established. That is why lemongrass is able to so actively eliminate disruptions in metabolism!

Lemongrass fruit tincture

Fruit tincture in 95% alcohol in a ratio of 1:5 is taken 20-30 drops 2-3 times a day to improve metabolism, as well as to activate the motor and secretory functions of the digestive organs.

Lemongrass seed powder

Schisandra seed powder (0.5-1 g 2-3 times a day) is used to improve metabolism, as well as to enhance visual acuity, accelerating the eye's adaptation to darkness.

Infusion of lemongrass berries

An infusion of 1 tablespoon of fresh or dried fruits per 1 cup of boiling water (infuse for 2 hours), take 2 tablespoons 4 times a day to improve metabolism.

Decoction of lemongrass berries

To improve metabolism, you need to drink a warm decoction of lemongrass berries: 20 g of berries per 1 cup of boiling water, leave for 30 minutes. Take 1 tablespoon 2-3 times a day.

lemongrass oil

Lemongrass oil speeds up the metabolism. It can be mixed with other oils that are shown to improve metabolism: grapefruit, ylang-ylang, fennel, juniper, ginger and take 1 teaspoon on an empty stomach in the morning. Schizandra oil is also used as a prophylactic for low blood pressure, fatigue and low performance, which are accompanied by lethargy and irritability; with disorders of the sexual sphere, the oil tones the cardiovascular system, improves vision and hearing, as well as other types of sensitivity; has an anti-inflammatory effect, improves digestion. It is a strong adaptogen.

Tonic salad

Such a salad will improve metabolism and give strength.

5 g lemongrass chinensis leaves

30 g nettle

30 g stonecrop

20 g dandelions

1 teaspoonLuke

1 tablespoon sunflower oil

50 g sour cream

Stonecrop large (hare cabbage) is a powerful stimulant that enhances regeneration and metabolic processes in tissues. This plant hasanti-inflammatory,

Lemongrass, raspberry, rosehip, currant leaves to activate metabolism

This infusion not only improves metabolism, but also prevents the development of fatigue.

1 part lemongrass leaves

1 part rosehip leaves

1 part raspberry leaves

1 part currant leaves

1 cup boiling water

Mix the crushed leaves of plants,

take 2 tablespoons of the collection, pour 1 cup boiling water in a thermos for 2 hours and take 1/2 cup 2 times a day.

fruit collection

An excellent remedy for eliminating disruptions in metabolism, forprevention of physical fatigue and increased mental tone.

1 part lemongrass berries

1 part cranberries

3 parts rose hips

1/2 l boiling water

100 g of the collection pour 1/2 liter of boiling water and boil for 10 minutes. The decoction is infused for 20 minutes. Then

strain and take 1/2 cup 2 times a day.

Lemongrass, ginger, wormwood and licorice

This tool improves metabolism and fights against the breakdown.

1 teaspoon lemongrass fruit

1 teaspoon wormwood

1 teaspoon aconite rhizome

1 teaspoon dry ginger

1 teaspoon licorice root

1 cup boiling water

Ignite the licorice root on fire, chop all the components, pour

1 cup boiling water, boil for 10 minutes, leave for 20 minutes.

Ginger is an amazing immunostimulant, multiplies strength, improves metabolism, improves tone, fights fatigue. The healing properties of ginger are enormous. It helps with almost all diseases.

Wormwood tones the stomach and improves digestion, it is shown as an analgesic, it is used for gout, rheumatism, bronchitis, pulmonary tuberculosis, anemia, nervous depression, exhaustion, impotence.

Licorice root strengthens the immune system, has anti-inflammatory, tonic, anti-allergic, antiviral, antitoxic, antibacterial, choleretic and diuretic effect, has a beneficial effect on the stomach.

Limonnikovo-nettle tincture

40 dry lemongrass berries

200 g May nettle

0.5 l of vodka or 50-60% alcohol

Pour crushed lemongrass berries and nettle leaves with vodka or alcohol, tie the dishes with gauze, stand the first day in the sun, then 8 days in a dark place, then strain the tincture. Drink 1 teaspoon 3 times a day 30 minutes before meals.

Lemon-nettle tea

2 teaspoons crushed lemongrass

2 heaping teaspoons minced nettle leaves and rhizomes

1/4 liter boiling water

I make tea like this: pour lemongrass and nettles with boiling water, boil for 5 minutes and filter. I drink warm, in small sips, 1 cup in the morning and in the evening for one to two months. This tea is good for metabolism.

Lemongrass and bran

50 g crushed lemongrass berries

crushed zest of one lemon

1 cup wheat bran

2 tablespoons honey

Pour all the ingredients into boiling water, bring to a boil. Let it brew for 1 hour, strain. Add honey and lemon juice. Drink warm 1/4 cup 2 times a day. You can prepare the infusion for 2-3 days and store in the refrigerator.

Drink from lemongrass berries with bran and blackcurrant

Can be used instead of blackcurrantuse raspberries or strawberries.

The drink normalizes metabolism and tones the body.

1.5 liters of water

1 cup wheat bran

50 g lemongrass berries

1 cup currant

2 tablespoons of sugar

15 g yeast

Squeeze juice from berries in a juicer. Boil pomace of berries in a small amount of water. Cool the broth, strain, combine with the resulting juice. Sift bran on a sieve, pour into boiling water, bring to a boil and insist for 1 hour. Strain, add yeast, mashed with sugar, to a decoction cooled to a temperature of 20-25 C. Leave for 2-3 hours to ferment at room temperature. Then add berry juice. Pour into a glass jar, close with a nylon lid and refrigerate for a day. The tonic drink is ready. It can be drunk cold and warm 2 times a day for 1/2 cup.

Lemongrass, horsetail and honey

2 tablespoons crushed lemongrass

100 g chopped horsetail herb

1 liter of water

- 250 g honey

I pour lemongrass berries and horsetail grass with water, cook in a sealed container over low heat until half of the liquid remains, then filter, squeeze, mix with honey and cook again - 30 minutes in a water bath, removing the foam. I store the medicine in a dark, cool place. It is necessary to take a decoction 3 times a day before meals, 1 tablespoon.

Horsetail is a powerful tool for improving metabolism. Horsetail cleanses the blood, removes toxins, removes excess cholesterol, removes lead.

Important:the plant is contraindicated in nephritis and nephrosis! For diseases of the gastrointestinal tract, it is necessary to take a drug that includes horsetail only after consulting a doctor!

Lemongrass, apples and squash

12 lemongrass leaves

1 kg young patissons

small apples

7 cherryleaves

7 blackcurrant leaves

1.5 liters of water

45 g sugar

15 g rye flour

25 g salt

Wash the squash with a brush, being careful not to damage the skin. Cut into 4 parts. Wash apples, cut, remove the core.

Put squash and apples in layers in a container (the height of the dishes should exceed its diameter), shifting with leaves of lemongrass, cherry, black currant. To pour, dissolve salt and sugar in boiling water, cool slightly and add toasted rye flour. Pour squash and apples, cover with boiled gauze folded in several layers, put a wooden circle with a load on top. Ferment in a cool place until the brine that has come out over the oppression stops foaming.

Lemongrass, beets, apples andplums

lemongrass leaves to taste

1 kg small young beets

700 g plums

small apples

1.5 l apple juice

cloves to taste

200 g sugar

20 g salt

Boil the beets until tender, peel. Clean the drainfrom bones.

Cut the apples in half and remove the core.

Cut beets, plums and apples into approximately the same circles. Blanch apples in boiling water for no more than 2 minutes. Put beets, plums, apples in layers in prepared jars and pour boiling filling of apple juice, sugar and salt with cloves and lemongrass leaves. Pasteurize and seal.

To improve metabolism, almost all recipes are suitable, which are given in the same chapter in the sections "To increase mental and physical endurance" and "To increase immunity."

Chapter 3 Treating with Lemongrass

With cardiovascular insufficiency

When using lemongrass preparations for cardiovascularinsufficiency, a doctor's recommendation is required.

There are many medicinal plants for the prevention of cardiovascular diseases and for their treatment. Lemongrass will help with non-organic diseases of the heart and blood vessels: with hypotension, vegetovascular dystonia of the hypotonic type, atherosclerosis, anemia.

With vegetovascular dystonia (VVD), malfunctions in the work of the autonomic nervous system occur, and it is this system that controls the balance in our body - heat exchange, blood circulation, digestion, the production of insulin and adrenaline. Tissues and organs receive less oxygen during VVD, we can feel attacks of dizziness, headache, pain in the heart area, rapid or slow heartbeat, shortness of breath, fever, lack of air, experience panic.

Sweating, weakness, weakness, fatigue, sleep disturbance, irritability, cold hands and feet are alsosymptoms of VSD. Lemongrass is great for correcting dystonia.

With vegetovascular dystonia of

the hypotonic type and hypotension

A tonic decoction of dried schisandra berries is very suitable for this disease.

10 g drylemongrass fruits

1 cup hotwater

Pour lemongrass with water, boil for 15 minutes, leave for 20 minutes, strain and bring to the original volume. Take 1 tablespoon morning and afternoon.

35-40 drops of lemongrass tincture three times a daybefore eating a good shop help with hypotension and atherosclerosis.

Lemongrass, rosehip and eight herbs for vegetovascular dystonia

1 part lemongrass fruit

5 parts rose hips

4 parts licorice root

3 parts valerian root

3 parts St. John's wort

2 parts mistletoe herb

2 parts angelica root

2 parts leuzea root

2 parts rhodiola root

1 part aralia root

1 liter of boiling water

Pour boiling water over 2 tablespoons of the pre-chopped

mixture, let it boil, boil over low heat for 10 minutes in a sealed container, pour into a thermos with the herb, insist overnight. Take the entire portion during the day, 100-150 ml half an hour before meals. The main dose (about 100 ml) should be taken in the morning. You can add honey, sugar or jam to taste. The course of treatment is 2 months.

With VVD (vegetovascular dystonia), herbalists recommend, in addition to alcoholic tincture of lemongrass, alcoholic tinctures from ginseng root - 3 times a day, 15-25 drops before meals, from zamaniha (the effect of zamaniha tincture is about the same as that of ginseng tincture) - with hypotension 30-40 drops 2-3 times a day before meals. The course of treatment is up to a month. Leuzea liquid extract is shown - 20-30 drops 2-3 times a day or Eleutherococcus liquid extract - 2 ml half an hour before meals for 2-4 weeks. With VSD, you need to sleep at least 8 hours a day. If it is difficult to fall asleep, you should drink hot milk with honey, lie down and relax all the muscles of the body. Proper nutrition is very important: vegetables, fruits, greens, cereals, sea fish. Less meat, sweet, strong coffee and tea, pickles, alcohol, eliminate nicotine. Try to eat more often those foods that contain a lot of potassium:eggplant, cabbage, apricots, prunes, potatoes.

Lemongrass with herbs for vegetovascular dystonia

2 parts lemongrass fruit

2 parts wormwood herb

2 parts dandelion root

2 parts knotweed herb

3 partsangelica root

3 partsfruits of viburnum

2 parts rose hips

2 parts aralia root

2 parts rhodiola root

2 partsleuzea root

2 partsnettle leaf

1 part coriander fruit

2 parts licorice root

1 liter of boiling water

Pour boiling water over 2 tablespoons of the pre-chopped mixture, let it boil, boil over low heat for 10 minutes in a sealed container, pour into a thermos with the herb, close tightly and leave overnight. Take the entire serving during the day, 0.5 cups half an hour before meals. You can add honey, sugar or jam to taste. The course of treatment is 2 months.

Lemongrass, mountain ash, hawthorn and multi-herbs with vegetovascular dystonia

2 parts lemongrass fruit

2 parts yarrow herb

2 parts licorice root

2 parts herb knotweed

2 parts knotweed herb

3 parts hawthorn fruit

2 partsrowan fruit

1 part aralia root

1 part rootLeuzei

2 parts stonecrop herb

1 part mordovnik root

2 parts tansy flowers

1 liter of boiling water

Pour boiling water over tablespoons of the pre-chopped mixture, let it boil, boil over low heat for 10 minutes in a sealed container, pour into a thermos with the herb, close tightly and leave overnight. Take the entire serving during the day, 0.5 cups half an hour before meals. You can add honey, sugar or jam to taste. The course of treatment is 2 months.

Hawthorn is a valuable food plant with excellent medicinal properties. Its softfloury fruits contain 5-10% sugars, mainly fructose, so they can be eaten with high blood sugar. Infusions of hawthorn fruits have a beneficial effect on the cardiovascular system, liver and gallbladder, and the gastrointestinal tract.

Hypotension is a frequent decrease in blood pressure.pressure below normal, that is, below 95/65 mmHg. Although there are people who feel good with 90/60 readings. If you systematically yawn day after day, you have heavy eyelids, weakness, fatigue, cold palms and feet, frequent headache, and even staggers when moving, and the temperature may be slightly lower, and at the same time the pressure is below normal, then you became hypotensive. Lemongrass is excellent at fighting this disease.

In the Far East, lemongrass is used even for hypertension - in the event that it is not accompanied by overexcitation of the nervous system and insomnia.

Lemongrass seeds for hypotension and vegetovascular dystonia Lemongrass seeds tincture not only increases blood pressure during

hypotension, but also restores

strength, stimulates mental and physical activity, strengthens the body as a whole, improves the functioning of the nervous and immune systems, as well as physical and psychological adaptation with a sharp change in external factors.

50 g lemongrass seeds

0.5 l vodka

Rinse the lemongrass seeds well to remove the remnants of the berry. Then they are thoroughly crushed and pour vodka. Place in a dark place for 14 days. The finished tincture is used 25 drops up to 3 times a day.

Lemongrass and black mulberry for hypotension

1 teaspoon chopped fresh or dried lemongrass

2 tablespoons chopped fresh or dry

1 cup boiling water

Pour boiling water over lemongrass and mulberry fruits, leave for 4 hours, strain. Drink a quarter cup 4 times a day before meals, but no later than 19 pm. Infusion cook once a day.

You can just eat lemongrass berries (no more than 5 berries a day) and mulberries: fresh - in summer, honey syrup from berries - in winter. Mulberry, like lemongrass, is healing all - and fruits, and bark, and leaves.

Schisandra tincture for low blood

pressure and vegetovascular dystonia

25 g lemongrass berries

100 ml alcohol

Pour lemongrass with alcohol, leave for 5-7 days in a dark place at room temperature, then strain. Drink 20-40 drops per 1 tablespoon of water before breakfast and lunch. The course is one month.

Lemongrass and stonecrop caustic for hypotension

1 teaspoon crushed lemongrass

20 g herb sedum

1 cup boiling water

Brew lemongrass and chopped

stonecrop herb with a glass of boiling water, leave for half an hour, strain. Take 1 tablespoon 3 times a day.

Stonecrop caustic helps not only with heart disease, but also with the stomach and liver.

Complex collection for hypotension: lemongrass, juniper, wild rose and a mixture of 10 herbs

1 part lemongrass fruit

1 part calamus roots

1 part juniper fruit

4 parts budra ivy herb

4 parts oregano herb

4 parts fireweed herb

4 parts plantain herb

2 parts verbena herb

2 parts gorse grass

2 parts peppermint herb

2 parts knotweed herb

6 parts rose hips

14 parts St. John's wort herb

0.5 l boiling water

Prepare a collection of crushedcomponents. Pour 2-3 tablespoons of the collection in the evening into a thermos and pour boiling water over it. Strain the next day. Drink 3 times a day 20-40 minutes before meals.

In addition to treatment with lemongrass or herbs, there are general recommendations - a contrast shower, a bath, a sauna (this is how we train blood vessels), good sleep, especially in the cold season, morning and afternoon coffee, strong sweet tea, green tea is especially good, regular meals during days - this is necessary for vascular tone. Juices are recommended for hypotensive patients, and a little red wine in the evening. Showing tinctures of ginseng, eleutherococcus, magnolia vine, Manchurian aralia immortelle. In addition, traditional healers recommend using cakes of cabbage, sorrel, plantain, cow parsnip.

Lemongrass and tartar with

hypotension

20 g drylemongrass fruits

30 g herb tartar

2 glassesboiling water

Pour boiling water over the crushed fruits and grass and insist overnight in a thermos. Take everything throughout the day 3 times before meals. The course is up to 3 weeks.

An infusion of herb tartar, as well as a powder from it, enhances heart contractions, eliminates palpitations, tones the body with hypotension and helps with heart weakness. Centuries ago, the Tatars certainly took bags with a Tatar man on campaigns. Before watering the horses or getting drunk themselves, they threw Tatar roots into the water, which purified the water so remarkably that it could be drunk without fear.

With atherosclerosis, lemongrass is also a faithful assistant. The disease lies in the fact that the vessels narrow or - which is much worse! -clogged. This is due to the formation of growths on their inner walls, the so-called plaques. The blood supply to all organs is deteriorating. If plaques are actively formed in the vessels going to the heart, this is fraught with a heart attack. If the arteries supplying the brain are affected, atherosclerosis can occur. Atherosclerosis kills!

But it is possible to significantly slow down the aging of blood vessels. It will help in this, in addition to the medication prescribed by the doctor, and the use of lemongrass.

Difficult collection for atherosclerosis:
lemongrass,hawthorn, wild rose and 12 herbs

1 part lemongrass fruit

2 parts hawthorn fruit

3 parts rose hips

2 parts budra ivy herb

2 parts Veronica officinalis herb

1 part sweet clover herb

1 part leaveswild strawberry

1 part red clover flowers

1 part raspberry leaves

1 part coltsfoot herb

2 parts dandelion roots

1 part plantain leaves

2 parts chamomile flowers

3 parts thyme herb

2 parts sage leaves

1 part mint leavespeppery

1 cup boiling water

Grind collection, mix. Pour boiling water over 1-2 tablespoons of the collection, leave for an hour, strain. Drink 3 times a day half an hour before meals. Infusion cook 1 time per day.

Lemongrass, sage and rose hips for

atherosclerosis

30 g crushed lemongrass

100 g chopped sage herb

100 g crushed rose hips

3 glassesboiling water

tablespoons of collection from the evening put in a thermos, pour boiling water. In the morning, strain and take 150 g 4 times a day 30 minutes before meals, but no later than 19 pm.

Infusion of lemongrass and lemon balm for atherosclerosis

1 tablespoon chopped lemongrass leaves

1 tablespoon chopped melissa herb

1 cup boiling water

Pour boiling water over lemon balm grass and lemongrass leaves, leave for 1 hour, strain. Take half a glass 4 times a day 30 minutes before meals, but no later than 19 pm.

Decoctions and infusions of lemon balm can be taken by everyone! Melissa treatment has no contraindications.

Lemongrass and hawthorn fruits for atherosclerosis

15g fresh or dried lemongrass

40 g fresh or dried hawthorn berries

2 glassesboiling water

Pour boiling water over the berries, leave for 2 hours, then bring to a boil and leave for another 1 hour in a warm place. Strain. Drink morning and evening 1 glass, but no later than 4-5 hours before bedtime.

Infusion of lemongrass and shepherd's purse for atherosclerosis

1 tablespoon chopped lemongrass leaves

1.5 tablespoons chopped shepherd's purse herb

450 g boiling water

Lemongrass leaves and shepherd's purse grass pour boiling water, leave for 1 hour, strain. Take 150 g 3 times a day.

Shepherd's purse is especially known for its hemostatic properties, as well as hypotensive and phytoncidal properties.

Limonnikovo-sage tincture for atherosclerosis

50 g chopped fresh or dried lemongrass

90 g chopped fresh sage herb

800 g vodka

400 g water

Mix lemongrass and sage herb with vodka and water. Infuse in the light for 40 days in a closed glass container. Take 1 tablespoon half and half with water in the morning before meals. The tincture is especially good for elderly people suffering from atherosclerosis. Course - 8 weeks.

With atherosclerosis, you need to

eat a lot of watermelons, onions, garlic, drink grapefruit juice. It is very good to eat a handful of walnuts a day. And not only admire the clover flowers, but also eat them - a lot!

lemongrass and threeherbs for atherosclerosis

10 g fruitslemongrass

20 g yarrow herb

20 g mistletoe

50 g Cystoseira bearded

1 cup boiling water

Brew 1 tablespoon of the crushed mixture with 1 cup of boiling water, insist, wrapped, 2 hours and strain. Drink everything in sips throughout the day. The course of treatment is 21 days.

White mistletoe well helps to normalize the work of the heart and blood vessels, nervous system, intestines, gives vitality, promotes weight loss.

Bearded cystorosis is an algae that improves metabolism and promotes weight loss.

Lemongrass and herbal collection for atherosclerosis

10 g fruitslemongrass

10 g rue herb

10 g goose cinquefoil

30 g mistletoe

30 g horsetail

1 glass of water

Pour 1 tablespoon of the crushed mixture with 1 glass of cold water, leave for 4 hours, boil for 4 minutes and strain. Drink everything in sips throughout the day. The course of treatment is 1 month.

Ruta is able to relieve spasms of smooth muscles of the digestive tract, biliary and urinary tract, as well as peripheralblood vessels, applied atdizziness, nervous diseases, pain in the stomach, relieves attacks of bronchial asthma, strengthens blood vessels and veins. Rue leaves have strong phytoncidal properties.

Potentilla improves immunity, normalizes the functioning of the thyroid gland, improves metabolism, and normalizes hormonal balance. Potentilla is used to treat diseases of the liver, cardiovascular system and gastrointestinal tract. This plant is an excellent blood purifier, antiseptic and wound healing agent.

Lemongrass, arnica, yarrow and St. John's wort in atherosclerosis

10 g fruitslemongrass

5 g mountain arnica

25 g yarrow herb

20 g St. John's wort

1 glass of water

Pour 1 cup of cold water with 1 tablespoon of the crushed mixture, leave for 2-3 hours, simmer for 5 minutes, leave for 15 minutes and strain. Drink everything in sips throughout the day. The course of treatment is 1 month. Arnica mountain has a stimulating effecteffect on the cardiovascular system, improves nutrition of the heart muscle, expandscoronary vessels, accelerates the heart rate, increases the amplitude of heart contractions, lowers blood cholesterol levels. Arnica is known asanti-inflammatory, choleretic hemostatic agent, reduces the excitability of the cerebral cortex and has a calming and anticonvulsant effect. One of the most common homeopathic plants.

John's wort is known for its anti-spasmodic properties,anti-inflammatory, diuretic, bactericidal, astringent, hemostatic and wound healing action, increases gastric secretion, treats gastritis, soothes.

Complex collection with lemongrass for atherosclerosis

10 g fruitslemongrass

10 g cumin fruit

10 g rue herb

10 g lemon balm herb

15 gvalerian root

20 g hawthorn flowers

20 g periwinkle leaves

30 g mistletoe herb

20 g fruitswild rose

1 cup boiling water

Brew 1 cup of boiling water 1 tablespoon of the crushed mixture and leave for 1 hour. Strain and drink all in sips throughout the day. The course of treatment is 1 month.

Lemongrass, lily of the valley, rue for atherosclerosis

10 g fruitslemongrass

10 g of May lily of the valley flowers

20 g lemon balm leaves

30 g goose cinquefoil herb

30 g rue herb

1 glass of water

Pour 1 glass of cold water with 1 tablespoon of the crushed

mixture, leave for 3 hours, simmer for 5 minutes, leave for 30 minutes and strain. Drink everything in sips throughout the day. The course of treatment is 1 month.

Lily of the valley is a heart remedy known in folk medicine: it enhances the contraction of the heart, improves blood circulation throughout the body, dilates the blood vessels of the kidneys, and calms the nervous system. Vfolk medicine, they have always been used to regulate cardiac activity, treat neurosis, tachycardia, etc.

Lemongrass with dandelion for atherosclerosis

1 tablespoon lemongrass fruit

3 tablespoons dandelion root

2 glassesboiling water

Boil the crushed fruits of lemongrass and dandelion roots with boiling water, bring to a boil and boil for 15 minutes over low heat. Drink 1 tablespoon 2 times a day 30 minutes before meals. Important: you need to dig up the roots of a dandelion either in early spring before flowering, or after the leaves wither. The course of treatment is 1 month.

Lemongrass leaves and buckwheat flowers in atherosclerosis

1 tablespoon chopped lemongrass leaves

1 tablespoon buckwheat flowers - fresh or dried

0.5 l boiling water

Pour lemongrass leaves and buckwheat flowers with boiling water, strain. You need to drink 1/2 cup 3 times a day. Infusion cook once a day.

Flowers and leaves of buckwheat are excellent for circulatory disorders, vasospasm and edema, with increased permeability and capillary fragility. Great remedy for atherosclerosisdiseases of the gastrointestinal tract and kidneys, anemia, disorders of the nervous system, bronchitis. Buckwheat is needed to improve metabolism in diabetes and obesity.

Lemongrass and periwinkle for atherosclerosis

10 g fruitslemongrass

30 g yarrow herb

15 g small periwinkle

15 g horsetail

15 g mistletoe

15 g hawthorn flowers

1 glass of water

Pour 1 cup of cold water with 1 tablespoon of the crushed mixture, leave for 1 hour, boil for 5 minutes, leave for 20 minutes and strain. Drink in sips throughout the day. The course of treatment is 3-4 weeks.

Periwinkle is used for the treatmentatherosclerosis, diseases

Infusion of lemongrass and thyme for atherosclerosis

1 teaspoon crushed lemongrass

1 teaspoon chopped thyme (thyme) herb

1 cup boiling water

Lemongrass fruit and thyme herbpour a glass of boiling water, insist, tightly closed and wrapped, 1 hour. Drink 1 tablespoon of infusion in the morning and evening. Infusion cook every day.

Thyme (thyme) able to remove

Lemongrass and soapwort in atherosclerosis

20 g fruitslemongrass

30 g dandelion roots

30 g wheatgrass

30 g soapwort

30 g yarrow herb

1 cup boiling water

Infuse 1 tablespoon of the crushed mixture in 1 cup of boiling water for 1 hour. Take 1 glass in the morning and early evening. The course of treatment is 3-4 months. soapwort is good for violations metabolism, for blood purification, in diseases of the liver and kidney,when coughing.

Wheatgrass improves metabolism, heals the body as a whole, cleanses of toxins, improves immunity, treats gastritis, helps fight stones in the gallbladder or bladder, is successfully used in the treatment of bronchitis, tracheitis, pneumonia - due to its expectorant properties, it is used as a diuretic and diaphoretic, as well as edema, provoked by heart disease.

Lemongrass tincture with the root of the step in atherosclerosis

25 g fruitslemongrass

50 g white foot root

0.5 l vodka

Insist lemongrass fruits and footstep roots in vodka for 10 days. Take 5 ml 3 times a day. The course of treatment is 3-4 weeks. Important: you can not use tincture for thrombophlebitis.

White step helps with pain in the heart, swelling of various origins, paralysis, epilepsy, intercostal neuralgia, diabetes. It has analgesic, antipyretic and anti-inflammatory effects.

Lemongrass and plantain in atherosclerosis

1 teaspoon crushed lemongrass

1 tablespoon dry crushed plantain leaves

1 cup boiling water

Pour boiling water over vegetable components and leave for 1 hour. Drink this daily dose in sips within an hour. The course of treatment is 3-4 weeks.

Basic nutrition in atherosclerosis should become nuts, vegetable oils, oily fish. These foods contain polyunsaturated fatty acids, and these acids can reverse the development of atherosclerosis, that is, significantly reduce the risk of heart attack and stroke. Fight against atherosclerosis biologically active substances flavonoids found in fresh vegetables and fruits. These substances are found in red wine, and in a number ofmedicinal herbs, for example, in ginseng, lemongrass, eleutherococcus, rhodiola rosea, skullcap, hawthorn.

In China and the Russian Far East, lemongrass fruits have long been used for anemia. Lemongrass increases the content of hemoglobin in the blood. You can drink a tincture or infusion of lemongrass berries, or you can combine lemongrass with other herbs.

Lemongrass and six herbs for anemia

1 part fresh lemongrass

4 parts lungwort roots

2 parts wild chicory roots

2 parts stinging nettle roots

4 parts rose hips

4 parts dandelion roots

2 parts plantain leaves

1 glass of water

2 tablespoons of the crushed mixture is poured with water, boiled over low heat for 10 minutes, insisted for 1 hour. Drink 50 ml 3 times a day 30 minutes before meals. The course is from one and a half to two months.

Lungwort contains many biologically activesubstances that

enhance blood formation. In addition, it perfectly cleanses the lungs and respiratory tract, stimulates the work of the endocrine glands, normalizes the immune system, and increases the protective properties of the body.

Chicory is used in sedative andhearty gatherings, where it serves as a wonderful addition to stronger herbs. Chicory improves the activity of the heart and blood vessels, prevents the formation of blood clots, strengthens the walls of blood vessels, improves immunity, has a sugar-lowering,astringent, choleretic, diuretic, anti-inflammatory action. Chicory removes toxins and heavy metals from the body. The main thingaction of chicory -

hepoprotective (restoring and improving liver function), so it is used as an adjuvant in diabetes mellitus.

Lemongrass and rosehipwith anemia

This remedy is also indicated for the normalization of metabolism and the good functioning of the gastrointestinal tract and kidneys.

1 tablespoon dry rosehip

1 teaspoon dried lemongrass berries

250 ml water

Lemongrass and rose hips should be brewed as tea and drunk 3 times a day after meals. The course is one month.

Lemongrass, currant, St. John's wort and clover for anemia

1 part lemongrass leaves

1 part currant leaves

1 part St. John's wort leaves

2 parts red clover

1 cup boiling water

Lemongrass should be brewed with herbs like tea and drunk 3 times a day after meals. The course is one month.

Red clover - increasesimmunity, strengthens and tones the body, has an anti-sclerotic effect, is indicated for anemia and beriberi. In addition, it has an expectorant, diuretic,choleretic, anti-inflammatory, antitoxic, wound healing, analgesic, hemostatic properties. Fights well any edema.

Lemongrass and mountain ash for anemia

2 teaspoons lemongrass fruit

2 teaspoons rowan fruit

2 glassesboiling water

Pour boiling water over chopped berries, leave for an hour and drink half a glass 3-4 times a day half an hour before meals. The course is one month.

Rowan is especially good for its effect on the circulatory and genitourinary systems. It also has a choleretic effect, lowers cholesterol, removes toxins from the body.

Lemongrass and three herbs for anemia

1 part crushed lemongrass

1 part minced nettle leaves

1 part crushed yarrow flowers

1 part chopped dandelion root

1.5 cups boiling water

Boil a tablespoon of the mixture with boiling water, leave for 3 hours, strain.Drink a day in 3-4 doses 20 minutes before meals. The course of treatment is 8 weeks.

For colds and respiratory diseases, influenza, bronchitis and tuberculosis

When using drugs for respiratory diseases, a doctor's recommendation is required.

Great for colds and respiratory problemsdecoctions of lemongrass leaves and bark. Lemongrass fruits perfectly increase the body's defenses, resistance to infections and reduce the likelihood of getting colds, flu and other diseases of the upper respiratory tract.

Herbal collection with lemongrass against colds and flu

3 partsnettle leaf

3 parts lemongrass shoots

1 part sage herb

1 cup boiling water

1 teaspoonhoney

Boiling water is poured into a thermos 1 teaspoon of crushed collection, insist 1-2 hours and drink after breakfast, adding honey. Sage enhances the action of lemongrass, and this property is often used in the countries of Southeast Asia - there it is valued no less than ginseng. Unfortunately, we usually use sage only for rinsing, forgetting about its excellent tonic properties.

A drop of lemongrass oil, applied to the sinuses, fights viral infections remarkably.

Berry-honey infusion for influenza and acute respiratory infections

1 teaspoon lemongrass fruit

1 tablespoon cinnamon rose hips

1 tablespoon dry blackcurrant berries

1 tablespoon dry raspberries

1 liter of boiling water

1 tablespoon honey

Take honey, lemongrass, rose hips, currant berries (variants are possible - currant jam, chopped dried leaves or sprigs of currant), raspberries (here, too, it is not necessary to take exactly berries - crushed dried leaves or twigs, jam, syrup will do). Pour boiling water over this mixture, wrap it up, insist for half an hour. Then strain. Drink half a glass several times a day. Every day prepare a new infusion.

Lemongrass,raspberries and honey for colds and flu

1 teaspoon dried lemongrass berries

2 tablespoons dried raspberries or raspberry jam

1 cup boiling water

1 tablespoon honey

Pour boiling water over dry berries of lemongrass, raspberries or raspberry jam, leave for 15 minutes, add honey and stir. It is better to drink this sweet medicine shortly before going to bed, as it has a diaphoretic effect. After drinking it and sweating, you need to wipe the body dry, change clothes, in no case get into a draft after treatment, do not drink cold drinks.

Lemongrass and currants for colds

1 tablespoon dried lemongrass berries

2 tablespoons dried berries or chopped blackcurrant sprigs

4 glassesboiling water

Pour dried berries of lemongrass and currants (or sprigs of black currant) with boiling water, boil over low heat for 5 minutes, wrap and leave for an hour. Strain and squeeze. Drink several times a day. In the evening before going to bed, you can add a little honey to this infusion. Every day prepare a new infusion.

Collection of herbs with lemongrass for colds

Very good for colds, in particular, increases sweating.

1 part crushed lemongrass

2 parts elderflower

2 parts flowerslindens

2 parts chamomile flowers

2 parts mullein flowers

2 parts blackthorn flowers

2 parts willow bark

1 cup boiling water

Brew a tablespoon of chopped raw materials with a glass of boiling water. Leave for 15 minutes, strain. Infusion drink hot 2-3 cups daily; each time prepare a new infusion.

Lemongrass, elderberry, chamomile for colds

1 part crushed lemongrass

2 parts chamomile flowers

2 parts black elderberry flowers

1 cup boiling water

Brew a tablespoon of chopped raw materials with a glass of boiling water. Leave for 15 minutes, strain. Infusion drink hot 2-3 cups daily; each time prepare a new infusion.

Chamomile is a well-known and very popular plant. Included in many herbal preparations for many diseases. Great for colds and asthma.

Infusion of lemongrass with four herbs for colds

1 part crushed lemongrass

2 parts chamomile flowers

2 parts black elderberry flowers

2 parts flowerslindens

2 parts mint leavespeppery

1 cup boiling water

Brew a tablespoon of chopped

raw materials with a glass of boiling water. Leave for 15 minutes, strain. Infusion drink hot 2-3 cups daily; each time prepare a new infusion.

Linden has excellent anti-cold properties: anti-inflammatory, diaphoretic and antipyretic. Therefore, with a cold, sore throat, tracheitis, bronchitis and pneumonia, it is difficult to find a replacement for lime.

Peppermint is also good for colds, as it has antibacterial and antispasmodic effects. In addition, mint will increase immunity and strengthen vitality, help the stomach and intestines, gallbladder, heart and blood vessels, with edema it is good as a diuretic, with insomnia - as a sedative. Acting as an antispasmodic, relieves headaches.

Anti-cold infusion

1 part crushed lemongrass

2 parts chamomile flowers

2 parts black elderberry flowers

2 parts flowerslindens

3 partsnettle leaf

1 part evasive peony flowers (marina root)

1 part licorice root

0.5 l boiling water

Brew 2 tablespoons of chopped collection with boiling water, leave for 15 minutes, strain. Infusion to drink warm during the day.

Peony improves efficiency, helps with insomnia, disorders of the nervous system and vegetative-vascular disorders, improves appetite and digestion, has a sedative, analgesic and bactericidal effect. The peony will also help with colds, in particular, with coughs.

Lemongrass will not be superfluous even if you have bronchitis. Atbronchitis infection penetrates deep into the bronchi. The main symptom of acute bronchitis is a cough, first dry, then wet, which can last up to two weeks. The temperature is usually low, unless, of course, bronchitis develops against the background of the flu. In this case, it can overshoot and over 39 C. Usually bronchitis is accompanied by a runny nose and pharyngitis. For centuries, bronchitis cough has been treated with plants.

Breast collection with lemongrass for bronchitis

Breast collection is called a set of medicinal herbs, a decoction of which helps to facilitate the removal of sputum (makes it more liquid), as well ashas an antimicrobial

1 part lemongrass fruit

1 part thyme herb (thyme)

1 part licorice root

1 part herb oregano

1 part Linden flowers

1 part peppermint herb

1 part coltsfoot herb

1 part plantain leaves

1 part pine buds

1 part herb lungwort officinalis

1 liter of boiling water for 4 tablespoons of chopped collection

Pour boiling water over 4 tablespoons of the crushed mixture of breast collection, wrap for an hour and a half. After insisting, strain and drink 150 g 4 times a day half an hour before meals.

Infusion of lemongrass and violet herb for chronic bronchitis

1 teaspoon crushed lemongrass

2 tablespoons chopped violet tricolor herb

2 glassesboiling water

Pour lemongrass and violet with boiling water and heat in a water bath for 15 minutes, leave for 45 minutes, strain, squeeze out the rest of the raw material. Bring the volume of the resulting infusion with boiled water to 2 cups. Take 0.5 cup 3-4 times a day. Every day prepare a new infusion.

Violet tricolor is an excellent expectorant. Indicated for coughs and colds; with catarrh of the upper respiratory tract, with bronchitis. It promotes liquefaction of sputum, its easier separation, has a diuretic and diaphoretic effect.

A decoction of lemongrass and five herbs for coughing

This decoction is recommended to drink when coughing,

1 part crushed lemongrass

1 part fenugreek seedshay

2 parts elderflower

1 part fennel fruit

2 parts grasstricolor violets

2 parts flowerslindens

1 glass of cold water

Insist a tablespoon of crushed collection in a glass of cold water for 2 hours, cook for several minutes and strain after cooling. Decoction drink warm in several doses in one day.

Lemongrass and oregano for treatmentbronchitis

Such a collection with lemongrass is a good expectorant.

1 part lemongrass fruit

1 part oregano herb

2 parts marshmallow root

2 parts coltsfoot leaves

2 glassesboiling water

Brew 1 tablespoon of chopped collection with boiling water, leave for 20 minutes, strain. Take 0.5 cup 3 times a day after meals.

Oregano is characteristicdiaphoretic, expectorant, diuretic, choleretic, anti-inflammatory, antiseptic, antispasmodic, and also calming effect.

Marshmallow officinalis has an expectorant, emollient and anti-inflammatory effect, enveloping the mucous membranes in case of diseases of the upper respiratory tract, stomach and intestines.

Coltsfoot is part of many chest collections, it treats bronchitis, laryngitis, tracheitis, pleurisy, bronchopneumonia, bronchial asthma, that is, it is remarkably good for all types of coughs and mucous sputum. In ancient Greece, when coughing, doctors advised to inhale the smoke from the burning leaves of the plant.

Lemongrass and nettle for the treatment of bronchitis

1 tablespoon lemongrass fruit

1 tablespoon nettle flowers

4 glassesboiling water

Lemongrass with nettle brew with boiling water, leave for half an hour, strainand drink 3-4 times a day an hour after meals.

Infusion of lemongrass and plantain for bronchitisThis infusion is good for bronchitis with viscous sputum.

1 tablespoon lemongrass fruit

4 tablespoons plantain leaves

0.5 cups boiling water

brewcrushed components with boiling water and insist 4 hours. Drink 1/2 cup 4 times a day half an hour after meals.

Lemongrass and ash for bronchitis

1 part lemongrass fruit

1 part ash leaves

1 part bark or young ash shoots

1 cup boiling water

It is necessary to pour 1 tablespoon of the crushed mixture with boiling water andheat over low heat for 20 minutes. Take 1 tablespoon 3 times a day half an hour after meals.

Ash tree – its leaves and bark – is used in folk medicine for the treatment of cough. A decoction of leaves and bark is used for bronchitis and bronchopneumonia, pulmonary tuberculosis, liver diseases, urolithiasis, inflammatory diseases of the kidneys, rheumatism, polyarthritis, sciatica, gout and dysentery, and also as an antihelminthic.

lemongrass and herbswith bronchitis and pneumonia

1 teaspoon lemongrass fruit

1 teaspoon herbknotweed

1 teaspoon coltsfoot leaves

1 teaspoon black elderberry flowers

1 cup boiling water

Brew the crushed components with a glass of boiling water, leave for 25-30minutes. Strain and drink 1/4 cup 4 times a day 30 minutes after meals.

Decoctions and infusions of knotweed herb haverestorative,

Lemongrass will also help with diseases such as pharyngitis and laryngitis. Pharyngitis is an inflammation of the mucous membrane of the pharynx. In acute pharyngitis, we feel dryness in the throat, pain when swallowing.Laryngitis is an inflammation of the larynx. It can occur from hypothermia, runny nose, acute respiratory infections, flu, and can also appear with prolonged voice tension. Dryness, sore throat, hoarseness, cough - first dry, then wet - are characteristic signs of laryngitis.

Lemongrass, sage, chamomile,

honey for pharyngitis

10 g Schizandra chinensis shoots

5 g sage

5 g chamomile

1 glass of cold water

Pour 10 g of crushed collection with water, boil for 2-3 minutes, leave for 2 hours. Take with warm honey 50 ml 2 times a day after meals.

Sage treats all inflammations in the nasopharynx and mouth, and chamomile - inflammatory processes not only in the nasopharynx and mouth, like sage, but also in the stomach.

Lemongrass, kefir,lemon and honey for pharyngitis

1 teaspoon lemongrass fruit decoction

250 ml kefir

1/2 lemon

1 teaspoonhoney

Make a decoction of lemongrass in the proportion of 1 part fruit to 20 parts water (boil for 15 minutes). Mix kefir, a teaspoon of broth, juice of half a lemon, honey. Take with sore throat 3-4 times a day after meals, 50 ml.

Lemongrass, rosehip, sageand honey for pharyngitis

50 ml decoctionlemongrass

100 ml sage infusion

50 ml rosehip infusion

15 g honey

Make a decoction of lemongrass (10 g per 200 ml), rosehip infusion (10 g per 200 ml) and sage infusion (5 g per 200 ml). Mix everything, add honey and take 200 ml once a day after meals at any time.

Infusion of lemongrass with dill for pharyngitis and laryngitis

1 teaspoon crushed lemongrass

1 tablespoon fennel seeds

1 cup boiling water

Pour lemongrass and dill with a glass of boiling water. Leave for 40 minutes, then strain. Drink a tablespoon 4-5 times a day. You can make an infusion for the whole day and use as needed throughout the day. This medicine is also an effective expectorant. Dill expectorant,bronchodilator,bactericidal,

antispasmodic,

Infusion of lemongrass and plantain leaves for pharyngitis and laryngitis This infusion is a good expectorant and anti-inflammatory

means. But for people with high acidity of gastric juiceany medicines and plantain dishes are strictly contraindicated!

1 teaspoon crushed lemongrass

3 teaspoons crushed plantain leaves

2 glassesboiling water

Lemongrass and plantain

pour boiling water. Insist half an hour. Then strain. Drink half a glass 3 times a day 20-30 minutes before meals. You can make an infusion for the whole day and use it throughout the day.

Lemongrass with sage and chamomile for pharyngitis and laryngitis

1 teaspoon crushed lemongrass

1 tablespoon chopped chamomile herb

1 tablespoon chopped sage herb officinalis Lemongrass and chamomile and sage herbs put in a thermos in the evening and

pour boiling water. Strain in the morning. Drink small amounts throughout the day.

Lemongrass and a variety of herbstracheitis

Lemongrass along with expectorants and mucus thinnersplants will accelerate recovery from tracheitis. You can mix the fruits of lemongrass with the leaves of the coltsfoot, licorice root, common yarrow herb, elecampane high, tripartite succession, thyme (common thyme), marshmallow root. Any plant that is used for infusion should be crushed beforehand.

1 teaspoon crushed lemongrass

2 tablespoons of any listed herb

0.5 l boiling water

Take a teaspoon of lemongrass and 2 tablespoons of any of these plants, pour boiling water, leave in a thermos for 2 hours, strain. Drink half a glass 3 times a day.

Important:infusion of lemongrass and licorice root drink 2 tablespoons 4 times a day.

Limonnikovo-anise infusion with angina

1 teaspoon crushed lemongrass

2 teaspoons crushed common anise

2 glassesboiling water

Pour the fruits of lemongrass and anise with boiling water, leave for an hour and strain. Drink a quarter cup 4 times a day. Every day it is recommended to prepare a new infusion.

Anise is useful for sore throats and coughs, ascharacterized

I think there is no person who has not had the flu or acute respiratory infections at least once in his life. Influenza spares no one during epidemics. But there is also herbal protection against influenza and acute respiratory infections. Teas from medicinal herbs - the more the better: thanks to them

flushes out the infection. Berries, fruits, vegetables that will strengthen the body. Infusions and decoctions of medicinal plants. And here lemongrass will provide effective help - both by itself and in a mixture with other medicinal plants.

Berry-honey infusion for influenza and acute respiratory infections

1 tablespoon lemongrass fruit

1 tablespoon cinnamon rose hips

1 tablespoon dry blackcurrant berries

1 tablespoon dry raspberries

1 liter of boiling water

1 tablespoon honey

Take honey, lemongrass fruits, rose hips, currant berries (variants are possible - currant jam, chopped dried leaves or currant twigs), raspberries (here, too, it is not necessary to take exactly berries - crushed dried leaves or twigs, jam, syrup will do). Pour boiling water over this mixture, wrap it up, insist for half an hour. Then strain. Drink half a glass several times a day. Every day prepare a new infusion.

Lemongrass and calamus for influenza and acute respiratory infections

This infusion is good for coughing and chest pain when coughing.

1 teaspoon crushed lemongrass

2 teaspoons crushed calamus leaves or roots

2 glassesboiling water

Pour boiling water over lemongrass fruits, leaves or roots of calamus, wrap for an hour (use a blanket, fur coat, etc.). Then strain. Drink a quarter cup 4 times a day. Every day prepare a new infusion.

Calamus tones and strengthens the body, helps with coughing, lowers blood pressure, has analgesic, expectorant, as well as antifungal and disinfectant effects.

Infusion of lemongrass with willow bark for influenza and acute respiratory infections

1/2 teaspoon crushed lemongrass

1/2 teaspoon chopped white willow bark or twigs

1/2 teaspoon crushed chamomile flowers

1/2 teaspoon crushed lime tree flowers

1/2 teaspoon crushed cinnamon rose hips

2 glassesboiling water

Schisandra berries, willow bark or twigs, chamomile and linden flowers,pour rose hips with boiling water, leave for 15 minutes, strain and squeeze. Drink a quarter cup 4 times a day. Every day prepare a new infusion.

Willow is a good helper in the treatment of colds, pleurisy, rheumatism, gout, gastritis, colitis, tachycardia, intestinal inflammation, diseases of the liver and spleen, and urinary tract. Rinse your mouth with a decoction of the bark for sore throat, stomatitis, gingivitis, periodontal disease. Bark baths are good for varicose veins.

Lemongrass can alleviate the patient's condition with pneumonia.In this disease, the tissues of the lungs become inflamed. Pneumonia is often the result of seasonal flu. In any form, pneumonia is a serious disease. Herbal treatment for pneumonia - as an addition to medication - is useful and healing.

35-40 drops of lemongrass tincture three times a day before meals will help as an adjuvant for pneumonia with vascular insufficiency and tuberculosis.

Lemongrass,herbs and pine for pneumonia

1 part lemongrass fruit

1 part thyme herb (thyme)

1 part knotweed grass

1 part anise fruit

1 part fragrant dill fruit

1 part licorice root

1 part pine buds

0.5 l boiling water

Prepare a mixture of plants - just equally. In the evening, take two tablespoons of the mixture, chop, pour into a thermos and pour boiling water over it. Insist until the morning. Strain. Drink half a glass of infusion 3 times a day. Every evening prepare a new infusion.

Pine needles have a beneficial effect on the cardiovascular system, slow down the aging process of the body, strengthen the immune system, and are also a good source of vitamins.

Lemongrass and three herbs for pneumonia

1 teaspoon lemongrass fruit

100 g herb primrose officinalis

75 g budry ivy herb

100 g comfrey root

3 glassesboiling water

Mix all ingredients. 3 tablespoons of crushed collection from the evening put in a thermos, pour boiling water. Strain in the morning. Take 150 g of infusion 4 times a day 30 minutes before meals. Every evening prepare a new infusion.

Primrose is an excellent vitamin andrestorative,
pneumonia. It is also indicated for anemia and spring beriberi, removes harmful substances from the body, relieves headaches, and helps with insomnia. Primrose regulates the functioning of the bladder and intestines, increases vitality.

Budra ivy treats bronchial asthma, pneumonia, diseases of the thyroid gland, gallbladder and liver. It is used in the treatment of skin diseases.

Comfrey root is used as an envelopinga remedy for all types of inflammation of the mucous membrane, and especially for pneumonia and other severe chest ailments.

With pneumonia, you need to drink tea from medicinalherbs: from thyme, lemon balm, rose hips, currants, raspberries, primrose, mint, sage, chamomile, oregano, linden, St. John's wort, strawberry leaves, lingonberry leaves, sweet clover, clover, tricolor violet, heather, elecampane. In any of these teas, you can add crushed lemongrass fruits - at the rate of 5 g per glass. You can add some honey to tea.

This tea flushes out bacterial toxins and antibiotics from the body. In addition, herbal tea is an excellent expectorant and antipyretic. It is important to remember that pneumonia requiresmandatory medical treatment. herbal medicine

- This is an additional method that can be added to the standard antibacterial. But not vice versa!

Tibetan medicine has been using lemongrass berries and seeds for centuries to treat tuberculosis, bronchial asthma, chronic bronchitis.

For these diseases, it is recommended to use:

Alcohol tincture of lemongrass (pharmacy or homemade): 20-30 drops with water on an empty stomach or 4 hours after eating;

Infusion of lemongrass (10 g of dry berries are infused in 1 cup of boiling water, taking 2 tablespoons on an empty stomach 2 times a day);

Lemongrass seed powder (0.5 g 2 times a day before meals).

All these drugs are takenno later than 4-5 hours before bedtime. Lemongrass, mistletoe and asparagus for tuberculosis

The mixture is shown not only as an aid in the treatmenttuberculosis, but also recommended for diabetes, anemia, loss of strength.

30 g powder fromlemongrass

fruits

150 g asparagus root powderlight

30 g mistletoe herb powder

some honey

Turn a mixture of powders with honey into pills and take 3-5 pieces 2-3 times a day.

With tuberculosis, bronchial asthma, bronchitis, Schisandra seed powder is useful - 1 g 3 times a day.

For diseases of the gastrointestinal tract, liver and kidneys

When using lemongrass preparations for the treatment of diseases of the gastrointestinal tract, liver and kidneys, a doctor's recommendation is required.

the digestive organs is the most directed. Decoctions, infusions and tinctures reach the digestive organs not indirectly, through the blood, but directly - irrigating and envelopingthe digestive tract from the tongue (it is also a digestive organ!) to the intestines. Therefore, the results of herbal treatment of the digestive tract do not have to wait long. Lemongrass skillfully helps with any gastritis, improves the motor and secretory functions of the gastrointestinal tract, has a beneficial effect on the functions of the liver and gallbladder, as well as kidneys, and simply improves appetite.

Lemongrass tincture to improve digestion

To improve digestionyou can take

a pharmacy tincture of lemongrass fruits in 95% alcohol in a ratio of 1:5. You need to drink 20-30 drops 2-3 times a day half an hour before meals. The course is one month. Such a medicine will improve the metabolism in general.

Doctors prescribe lemongrass for any gastritis. Gastritis is an inflammation of the lining of the stomach. Symptoms of acute gastritis include heaviness and overflow in the stomach, nausea, often accompanied by vomiting and diarrhea. Chronic gastritis is also characterized by pressure and distension "in the pit of the stomach" after eating, heartburn, loss of appetite, dull pain, sour belching. Sometimes gastritis is accompanied by constipation, and often by night pains.

Acute gastritis should be diagnosed by a doctor, self-treatment of abdominal pain is unacceptable!

The main treatment for gastritis is a proper diet: eating up to 6 times a day in small portions. As an additional treatment

Lemongrass is perfect.

It is only necessary to know the specifics of the impact of individual parts of the plant on the human body. In particular, the juice is used effectively with low acidity of gastric juice, and seed powder - with high acidity. In collections with herbs with increased acidity of gastric juice, crushed lemongrass fruits are often used.

With gastritis, which is accompanied by an increase in the acidity of gastric juice, it is recommended to regularly take powder from the seeds of lemongrass: 0.5-1 g 2-3 times a day.

With gastritis with low acidity of gastric juice, regular intake of juice from lemongrass berries gives a good effect: one tablespoon 3 times a day before meals.

Lemongrass collection of six herbs in gastritis

1 tablespoon lemongrass berries

1 tablespoon black elderberry flowers

1 tablespoon chamomile flowers

0.5 tbsp fennel fruit

0.5 tablespoon of inflorescences with bracts of linden cordifolia

1 tablespoon melissa herb

1 tablespoon peppermint herb

1 cup boiling water

Pour a tablespoon of the mixture with a glass of boiling water, soak for 10 minutes on low heat in a sealed container, leave for 2 hours, strain. Take 1-3 - 1-2 cups three times a day 1 hour after meals.

Lemongrass, herbs and honey for the normal functioning of the gastrointestinaltract

15 g fruitslemongrass

15 g dill fruits

15 g plantain leaves

10 g fruitswild rose

10 g St. John's wort

5 g flax seeds

5 g wormwood herb

5 g chamomile flowers

0.5 l boiling water

1 tablespoon of honey per glass of decoction

You need to take two tablespoons of crushed dry mixture and pour boiling water over it. After that, simmer for a coupleminutes. Infuse for 1 hour, and then dissolve bee honey in it. Drink 0.5 cup 4 times a day 2 hours before meals.

Herbal lemongrass decoction with increased acidity of gastric juice

15 g fruitslemongrass

10 g peppermint herb

10 g small-leaved linden flowers

20 g marsh rootcalamus

20 g licorice root

20 gfennel fruit

20 g flax seeds

0.5 l boiling water

1 tablespoon of honey per glass of decoction

You need to take two tablespoons of crushed dry mixture and pour boiling water over it. After that, boil on low heat for 15 minutes. Infuse for 1 hour, strain, and then dissolve bee honey in it. Drink 0.5 cup 3 times a day for an hour and a half before meals.

Traditional medicine includes fennel in recipes for decoctions that eliminate flatulence, cough, insomnia, abdominal pain, and increase lactation.

In official medicine, fennel is used as an aid in the treatment of bronchitis, bronchial asthma, pulmonary tuberculosis, urinary tract infections, gastritis, hepatitis, colitis, pharyngitis, and stomatitis.

Fennel has a beneficial effect on the cardiovascular system, is useful for angina pectoris, coronary heart disease, vegetovascular dystonia.

Important:women should use fennel with caution in diseases of the gynecological sphere. Fennel consumption may causeuterine bleeding in the first weeks of pregnancy.

Lemongrass with herbs and honey for acute gastritis

15 g fruitslemongrass

20 g yarrow herb

20 g chamomile flowers

20 g plantain leaves

20 g herb tripartite

0.5 l boiling water

All these components are

necessarychop and pour boiling water, then keep on low heat for another 3-4 minutes. Then let the collection brew for 30 minutes, strain and dissolve 1 tablespoon of honey in it. In acute gastritis, it is recommended to take half a glass of decoction 3 times a day one hour before meals.

The succession has a diuretic, diaphoretic, antipyretic, anti-inflammatory and anti-allergic effect, improves metabolism.

Infusion of lemongrass and rose hips to improve the functioning of the digestive system and liver

This infusion hasexcellent choleretic, wound healing and anti-inflammatory action. It is indicated for gastritis, inflammation of the liver and biliary tract.

1 part lemongrass fruit

1 part rose hips

40 parts water

Pour the fruits with boiling water and insist2 hours. Strain. Take half a glass 3 times a day 30 minutes before meals.

Lemongrass and calendula to improve the functioning of the digestive system and liver

This decoction of calendula has on the bodyanti-inflammatory, choleretic, disinfectant and astringent action.

2 teaspoons crushed lemongrass

2 tablespoons of calendula flowers

0.5 l water

Pour the ingredients with boiling water and put on a slow fire. Bring the broth to a boil and leave for 2 hours. Strain and take 1/4 cup 3-4 times a day.

Calendula will come to the rescue with cholecystitis, gastritis, colitis, hepatitis, stomach ulcers andduodenum, as well as hypertension and angina pectoris, atrial fibrillation and neurosis, thrombophlebitis and laryngitis, stomatitis and cervical erosion.

Lemongrass and sage for gastritis and enterocolitis

1 part lemongrass fruit

1 part sage leaves

60 parts water

Pour the crushed components with boiling water and leave for 2 hours.

Take 1/4 cup 3 times a day 30 minutes before meals.

A few general recommendations: with increased acidity of gastric juice, you need to drink carrot juice or a mixture of potato and carrot juices (up to 100 ml on an empty stomach). Potato juice neutralizes the acid. Walnuts reduce acidity, they need to be eaten 8-15 pieces per day.

Lemongrass and plantain with low gastric acidity

1 part berry juicelemongrass

1 part plantain juice

1 part honey

Mix the ingredients, store the mixture in a cool place. Take 1 dessert spoon 2-3 times a day 10 minutes before meals.

Lemongrass and wormwood with low acidity of gastric juice

1 tablespoon lemongrass juice

1 teaspoon wormwood

1 cup boiling water

a teaspoon of wormwood pour a glass of boiling water. Cool down. Add lemongrass juice. Take 1 tablespoon 3 times a day 15-20 minutes before meals.

Lemongrass with hops for inflammation of the liver, gallbladder and kidneys

Such an infusion is also suitable

for other inflammatory processes in the gallbladder and liver, as well as in the kidneys.

10 g fruitslemongrass

10 g hops

1 cup boiling water

Brew a glass of boiling heels with a mellow or lemongrass, insist 1hour, strain. Take 1 tablespoon 3 timesa day half an hour before meals.

Hops are very good for the gastrointestinal tract in general. In addition, it will help with vegetovascular dystonia, nervous disorders, skin diseases, restore sleep and reduce the symptoms of menopause.

Five-herbal collection with

lemongrass for the liver and gallbladder

15 g fruitslemongrass

15 g mint leaves

2 g bean

15 g yarrow flower baskets

15 g dill seeds

30 g St. John's wort

2 glassesboiling water

tablespoons of the crushed mixture are poured with boiling water, insist

2 hours, filter and take during the day the entire portion of 1-2 tablespoons per reception half an hour before meals.

Lemongrass and budra ivy for the liver and gallbladder

1 teaspoon lemongrass fruit

1 teaspoon budra ivy

1 cup boiling water

Brew the crushed components with 1 cup of boiling water, leave for 1 hour, wrapped, and strain. Drink 1/3 cup 3 times a day 30 minutes before meals.

Lemon-birch infusion for the liver

It is used for cholecystitis and hepatitis, as well as to relieve edema caused by heart failure.

1 teaspoon crushed lemongrass

2 teaspoons chopped spring birch leaves

1 cup boiling water

Boil fruits and leaves with boiling water and leave for 1 hour. Strain.

Take 1/3 cup 3 times a day half an hour before meals.

Birch leaves are used for cholecystitis, rheumatism, sciatica, a decoction of them is an excellent diuretic and disinfectant.

Lemongrass and mint for the gallbladderUsed as a choleretic agent.

1 teaspoon lemongrass fruit

1 teaspoon peppermint herb

1 cup boiling water

Pour boiling water over crushed fruits and grass, heat for 15 minutes in a water bath. Strain and drink 1/3 - 1/2 cup 2-3 times a day half an hour before meals.

Lemongrass and oregano for the gallbladder

This infusion is used to treat biliary tract.

1 teaspoon lemongrass fruit

1 teaspoon herboregano

1 cup boiling water

Pour lemongrass and oregano with boiling water, leave for 2 hours and strain.

Drink 1/4 cup 3 times a day half an hour before meals.

Lemongrass and herbal collection for cholecystitis

1 part lemongrass fruit

3 parts St. John's wort

2 parts wormwood herb

2 parts peppermint

2 parts valerian root

1 part hop cones

1 liter of boiling water

5 tablespoons choppedcollection pour boiling water and boil in a water bath for 15 minutes. Leave for 1 hour and strain. Drink 1-2 glasses 2-3 times a day 30 minutes before meals. As an additional component, you can use powder from immortelle flowers or chicory roots (on the tip of a knife).

Valerian calms, has a beneficial effect on the cardiovascular system and the gastrointestinal tract. It will relieve pain in the liver, expandcoronary vessels of the heart, has an antispasmodic effect, normalizes blood circulation.

Lemongrass and cumin to enhance pancreatic function

1 teaspoon crushed lemongrass

1 tablespoon cumin

1 cup boiling water

Put the components in a thermos, pour a glass of boiling water. Strain in the morning, divide into 4 doses and take 4 times a day one hour before meals.

About cumin, the prophet Muhammad said that he "heals

everything except death." Cumin increases protectiveproperties of the body, expands the bronchial passages, regulates blood pressure, prevents vasospasm, enhances the secretion of bile. With regular taking black cumin normalizes the contentcholesterol. Seeds and black cumin oil lower blood sugar in diabetic patients, have a positive effect on blood hemoglobin levels in anemia. In homeopathy, black cumin seed tincture is used to treat diseases of the gastrointestinal tract.

Lemongrass and rose hips for the kidneys and stomach

This remedy will also help with anemia, scurvy, and metabolic disorders.

- 2 heaped teaspoons of dry rose hips
- 1 teaspoon dried lemongrass berries
- 250 ml water

Lemongrass and rose hips should be brewed as tea and drunk 3 times a day after meals. The course is one month.

With inflammation of the kidneys, it is desirable

Lemongrass and bearberry for nephritis

The infusion is used for acute and chronic nephritis.

- 1 teaspoon lemongrass fruit
- 1 tablespoon bearberry (bear's ear)
- 1 cup boiling water

Pour the chopped ingredients with 1 cup of boiling water and leave, wrapped, for 30 minutes. Strain and drink 4-5 times a day, 1 tablespoon 30 minutes after eating. Important: the infusion should not be used for glomerulonephritis and pregnancy.

Bearberry is an excellent diuretic, cleanses the kidneys and blood, normalizes metabolism, and is used for nervous disorders.

Lemongrass and bedstraw with nephritis

It is used for nephritis, pyelitis, pyelonephritis.

1 teaspoon lemongrass fruit

1-2 teaspoons of real bedstraw herb

1 cup boiling water

Pour boiling water over chopped fruits and herbs, keep in a water bath for 15 minutes, leave for 30 minutes and strain. Drink 1-2 tablespoons 4-5 times a day 30 minutes before meals.

In folk medicine, the bedstraw has long been used to treat liver and kidney diseases, digestive disorders, eczema and scurvy. In addition, the bedstraw is indicated for nervous instability, insomnia.

Lemongrass and four herbs for nephritis

This decoction is especially good for chronic nephritis.

1 part lemongrass fruit

1 part lovage root

1 part steel root

1 part licorice root

1 part juniper fruit

1 cup boiling water

Pour 1 cup of boiling water over 1 tablespoon of the chopped mixture, leave for 6 hours, boil for 15 minutes and strain. Drink in several doses after meals. Important: the decoction should not be drunk during pregnancy and acute inflammation of the kidneys.

Lovage is a very famous herb. It has excellent diuretic properties, has a good effect on the heart and blood vessels, tones and strengthens the body, has antimicrobial and anti-inflammatory effects. Help with various diseases of the upper respiratory tract, as well as nervous disorders, problems with the gastrointestinal tract, gout and rheumatism. Since ancient times, lovage leaves have helped get rid of migraines - they were simply applied to the head.

Field stalnik is an anti-inflammatory herb. It has a diuretic effect, good for bladder stones. Perfectly helps with hemorrhoids, strengthens blood vessels, cleanses the blood.

Juniper is a plant revered since biblical times, which has bactericidal, antiseptic and anti-inflammatory effects. Volatile secretions of juniper kill a third of the microbes contained in the air.

Lemongrass, juniper, fennel and licorice for jade

15 g fruitslemongrass

60 g juniper fruit

20 g fennel seeds

20 g licorice root

1 cup boiling water

Pour 1 cup of boiling water over 1

tablespoon of the chopped mixture, heat over low heat for 20 minutes, leave for 30 minutes and strain. Drink 1 day in divided doses after meals. Important: the infusion should not be used during pregnancy and acute inflammation of the kidneys.

Lemongrass and herbal collection for nephritis

This infusion is good for chronic nephritis.

15 g fruitslemongrass

25 g piculnik herb

25 g horsetail herb

50 g knotweed herb

1 glass of water

Pour 1 tablespoon of the crushed mixture with 1 glass of cold water, leave for 6 hours, then boil for 5 minutes over low heat and strain. Drink 1-2 glasses a day after meals.

Pikulnikovpossesses tonic, diuretic, blood-purifying action. Good for diseases of the kidneys and gallbladder.

Lemongrass,flax, harrow and birch leaves with jade

20 g fruitslemongrass

40 g flaxseed

30 g harrow root

30 g white birch leaves

1 glass of water

Pour 1 tablespoon of the crushed mixture with 1 glass of cold water, leave for 6 hours, then boil for 5 minutes over low heat and strain. Drink 1/3 cup 3 times a day after meals.

Flax seeds are unique in their healing properties. They are used for any inflammation, for diseases of the heart and blood vessels, for oncological diseases, for diabetes, they purify the blood, strengthen the immune system.

Lemongrass, juniper and quince with jadeThis drink will help with chronic nephritis.

10 g fruitslemongrass

30 g juniper fruit

30 g whole quince seeds

1 cup boiling water

Pour boiling water over the mixture, put on fire, bring to a boil and heat on a low flame for 20 minutes, then leave for 1-2 hours and strain. Drink in several doses after meals.

Quince seeds treat diseases of the kidneys, stomach, constipation, and are also used as an expectorant. Important: the seeds cannot be crushed, if when crushed, they release the poisonous substance amygdalin, which gives the quince the smell of bitter almonds.

Lemongrass, birch and dandelion for jade

10 g fruitslemongrass

10 g juniper fruit

10 g white birch leaves

10 g dandelion root

1 cup boiling water

Pour 1 cup of boiling water over 1 tablespoon of the chopped mixture, leave to cool and strain. Drink 3 times a day, 1 tablespoon after meals.

Diuretic collection with lemongrass for inflammation of the kidneys

Such an anti-inflammatory, antimicrobial and diuretic collection is indicated for inflammation of the kidneys.

1 part lemongrass berries

1 part comfrey root

1 part St. John's wort

1 part violet herbtricolor

1 part herbmotherwort

1 cup boiling water

Boil 10 g of the crushed mixture with 1 cup of boiling water, soak for 15 minutes in a water bath and leave for 30 minutes. Then strain and drink 1/3 cup 3 times a day after meals.

Lemongrass and hernia in diseaseskidney

1 teaspoon lemongrass fruit

3 teaspoons dried herb sweet herb

1 cup boiling water

Brew the chopped mixture with 1 cup of boiling water, boil for 5 minutes and leave for 30 minutes. Drink 1 tablespoon 5-6 times a day.

Gryzhnik sweet is an excellent medicine for any kidney disease, especially for acute nephritis, acute inflammatory processes and spasms of the bladder. It is used only in traditional medicine.

Lemongrass and cuff for kidney disease

2 teaspoons lemongrass fruit

3 tablespoons of common cuff

2 glassesboiling water

Pour boiling water over the crushed mixture, insist, wrapped, 4 hours and strain. Drink 1/2 cup 3-4 times a day 30 minutes before meals.

The cuff, which is also called an ailing herb, has not only a diuretic, but also a strong anti-inflammatory effect, so it is excellent for kidney and bladder diseases, chronic intestinal inflammation, gastritis and stomach ulcers, inflammatory diseases of the upper respiratory tract, tuberculosis, bleeding, female diseases .

Golden infusion with lemongrass for inflammation of the kidneys

This infusion is an excellent anti-inflammatory and

1 part lemongrass berries

1 part comfrey root

1 partgolden rod herbs

0.5 l water

Pour boiling water over 2 tablespoons of the chopped mixture, insist overnightin a thermos and strain. Drink 1/2 cup 2-3 times a day after meals.

The herb golden rod is known as a wonderful remedy for chronic kidney disease, enterocolitis and cholelithiasis.

Lemongrass and flaxseed for kidney disease

1 teaspoon lemongrass fruit

1-2 tablespoons of herbs and flowersflaxseeds

1 cup boiling water

Brew 1 cup boiling water 1-2 tablespoonsspoons of the crushed mixture, leave for 30 minutes and strain. Drink 1-2 tablespoons every 1-2 hours.

Flaxseed - snapdragon - treats the kidneys, bladder, biliary tract, constipation, hemorrhoids, is used for hypertrophy and inflammation of the prostate gland, for shortness of breath, hypertension, palpitations, intestinal atony.

Infusion of lemongrass with aspen bark for kidney disease

1 teaspoon lemongrass fruit

1 tablespoon of kidney or aspen bark

1 cup boiling water

Pour 1 cup of boiling water over the crushed fruits of lemongrass and buds or dried and chopped bark of a young aspen tree, boil over low heat for 15 minutes, leave for 30 minutes and strain. Drink 2 tablespoons 3-4 times a day 30 minutes before meals.

An infusion or decoction of aspen bark or buds is used for kidney diseases, urinary retention, cystitis, prostate hypertrophy and other diseases of the bladder, for disorders of the gastrointestinal tract, rheumatism, gout, hemorrhoids.

Limonnikovo-birch infusion for kidney disease

20 g fruitslemongrass

100 g white birch leaves

2 glasseswater

Pour crushed lemongrass fruits and young spring birch leaves with 2 cups of warm boiled water and insist overnight in a thermos, then strain and squeeze out the remainder. Drink 1/2 cup 2-3 times a day 15-20 minutes before meals. traditional Chinese medicine uses lemongrass for urinary incontinence and diarrhea.

For men's health problems

When using lemongrass preparations to improve malehealth, a doctor's recommendation is required.

Lemongrass tincture is especially indicated for disorders in the genital area associated with chronic adrenal insufficiency. In Chinese medicine, lemongrass belongs to the first category of medicinal products. According to ancient Chinese treatises, lemongrass

"prevents the disappearance of energy and gives shine to the eyes." Lemongrassin its pure form or mixed with other plants, doctors recommend for infertility and impotence. In its pure form, for the treatment of these diseases, lemongrass is used as a tincture and as an infusion.

Lemongrass tincture for sexual weakness

It is necessary to take pharmacy or homemade lemongrass tincture 20-30 drops 2-3 times a day before meals for a month, but no later than 5 hours before bedtime.

Lemongrass infusion for sexual weakness

10 g crushed lemongrass

1 cup boiling water

Pour boiling water over

lemongrass, leave for 6 hours and take 1 tablespoon 2 times a day for a month, but no later than 5 hours before bedtime.

You can use fresh or dry leaves instead of fruits - 1 teaspoon of crushed leaves per 1 cup of boiling water.

You can eat 2-5 fresh fruits or 0.5 g of powder 2 times in the first half of the day to enhance potency.

Lemongrass with herbs for sexualweaknesses

15 g dried lemongrass

20 g yarrow herb

30 g herb oregano

30 g rootselecampane

40 g St. John's wortor highlander bird

1 cup boiling water

All components are crushed and mixed. Pour 1 cup of boiling water over 1 teaspoon of the mixture, insist until cool and filter. Take 1/4 cup 4 times a day. The course of treatment is 2 weeks.

Elecampane improves metabolism, is used in violation of the gastrointestinal tract and as a diuretic, removes heavy metals, radionuclides, toxins from the body, lowers cholesterol levels.

Highlander bird hasanti-inflammatory, antimicrobial, diuretic properties, accelerates wound healing, improves immunity, reduces the crystallization of mineral salts in the urinary tract.

Lemongrass and four herbs to enhancepotency

3 teaspoons lemongrass fruit

5 teahousesspoons of mint

5 teaspoons clover

5 teaspoons St. John's wort

5 teaspoons nettle

1 liter of boiling water

Mix the crushed ingredients, pour the mixture with boiling water and insist in a thermos for 20 minutes. Strain and drink 1 glass 3-4 times a day. The course of treatment is 2-3 weeks.

Lemongrass and St. John's wort

for men

This infusion is recommended for impotence.

1 teaspoon lemongrass fruit

1 tablespoon St. John's wort with flowers

1 cup boiling water

Pour the crushed components with boiling water, leave for 30 minutes, strain and take 1/2 cup 3 times a day.

Six tinctures to enhance potency

It is necessary to mix 30 ml of lemongrass tincture, 50 ml of aralia tincture, 50 ml of ginseng tincture, 50 ml of lure tincture, 30 ml of Rhodiola rosea extract and 30 ml of Eleutherococcus extract.

Drink 30 drops of the mixture 3 times a day after meals.

Lemongrass and yarrow for sexual weakness

10 g fruitslemongrass

100 g yarrow herb

50 g calamus root

50 g fenugreek seeds

1 cup boiling water

Mix the ingredients, pour boiling water over 1 tablespoon of the chopped mixture, leave for 1 hour, strain. Drink 3 cups of infusion per day.

Hay fenugreek - mushroom grass, trigonella,fenugreek, Greek shamrock, cocked hat, camel grass, chaman, shamballa. Grass seeds are good for sexual weakness, chronic cough, anemia, enlarged liver and spleen, gout, diabetes, neurasthenia, and also have a good diuretic effect. The ancient Egyptians used fenugreek seeds to embalm mummies. A number of scientists consider hay fenugreek to be a powerful stimulant and an effective medicine for eliminating metabolic failures.

Lemongrass and periwinkle for problems with potency

10 g fruitslemongrass

20 g herbs and periwinkle flowers

1 cup boiling water

Brew lemongrass and periwinkle with boiling water, cook for 5 minutes over low heat and leave for 30 minutes. Drink 8 drops in the morning and evening for 4 days, then take a break for 2 days and again conduct a four-day course. Continue taking drops intermittently until the entire decoction is used.

Periwinkle will improve metabolism, help with sexual weakness, peptic ulcer of the stomach and esophagus, vegetovascular dystonia, bronchitis, colitis, enteritis, migraine.

Lemongrass with hawthorn to enhance potency

10 g fruitslemongrass

15 g rue herb

25 g hawthorn leaves

25 g hawthorn flowers

10 gvalerian root

1 glass of cold water

Mix the ingredients, pour 1 tablespoon of the crushed mixture with water, leave for 3 hours, then boil for 4 minutes, leave for 20 minutes and strain. Drink in sips for 1 day. The course of treatment is 3-4 weeks.

Love Potion with Lemongrass

1 teaspoon crushed dry lemongrass leaves

1 tablespoon ground coffee

1 cup hotwater

Mix lemongrass and coffee, add

water and, stirring slowly, bring to a boil. Remove from heat, let steep for 5 minutes. Strain, sweeten slightly and drink 2 times a day. The course is one month.

Lemongrass and motherwortprostatitis

This infusion relieves inflammation, helps restore normal urination.

15 g lemongrass fruits

20 g rose hips

40 g motherwort herb

20 g plantain leaves

20 g birch leaves

0.5 l boiling water

Grind each component, mix

everything. 3 tablespoons pour the dry mixture with boiling water in a thermos. Infuse for 3 hours, then strain. In the resulting infusion, add honey to taste. Take the infusion warm in half a glass 3 times a day half an hour before meals. It is best to drink it for a month, then take a break for 3 weeks and repeat the treatment.

Motherwort calms,

Lemongrass and a variety of herbs for prostatitis

It is used for prostatitis and prostate adenoma.

1 part lemongrass fruit

1 part chamomile flowers

1 part marigold flowers

1 part yarutka herb

1 part knotweed herbavian

1 part sweet clover grass

1 part sage herb

1 part mistletoe herb

1 part horsetail

1 part Veronica officinalis herb

1 parthazel leaf

1 part coltsfoot herb

1 part chicory root

1 part rose hips

1 part aspen bark

1 cup boiling water

Pour boiling water over 1 tablespoon of chopped collection, soak in a water bath for 15 minutes, leave for 30-40 minutes, strain. Drink 0.5 cup 3 times a day before meals.

Yarutka increases potency and also hasantibacterial, vitamin, wound healing, expectorant, diuretic, astringent, tonic properties.

Sweet clover relieves inflammation, a good antispasmodic, in addition, it has a narcotic, hypotensive, expectorant, analgesic, wound healing, diuretic effect.

Veronical medicinal

The leaves and bark of hazel are an excellent anti-inflammatory agent. They are used to treat intestinal diseases and the liver, constricts blood vessels.

Coltsfoot not only helps with coughing, but is also an excellent diuretic used for inflammation of the bladder and urinary tract, kidneys, and edema. This herb is also good for diseases of the stomach and other organs of the gastrointestinal tract.

Lemongrass and hernia naked

with prostatitis

2 teaspoons lemongrass fruit

4 tablespoons hernia

1.5 cups boiling water

Pour the crushed components with boiling water, leave for 2 hours, strain and store in the refrigerator. Drink 1 tablespoon 3-4 times a day before meals. The course is 21 days, a week is a break.

Lemongrass and wintergreen - a remedy for prostatitis

1 teaspoon lemongrass fruit

1 tablespoon wintergreen herb

1 cup boiling water

Pour the crushed mixture with

boiling water, insist in a dark place for 3 hours, strain, drink 50 g 3 times a day before meals. Course - 1 month.

For men

A mixture of three tinctures for prostate adenoma

200 g aspen bark

0.5 l vodka

1 l redberry

1 liter of vodka

1 l lemongrass clusters

0.5 l alcohol

At the beginning of summer, when sap is still flowing, it is necessary to prepare the bark of young aspens. You need to remove the bark with a tube. Dry (you can in the oven, but not in the sun), cut into pieces of 2-3 cm and pour vodka. Close tightly and put in a dark place for 15-20 days. Then strain the tincture and put in a dark place. At the end of summer whenwild berries ripen, you need to take 1 liter of freshly harvested Far Eastern redberry (bugs) and pour 1 liter of vodka into it. Insist in a dark place for 2 weeks, strain, squeeze the berries. Next, pour lemongrass berries with pure alcohol. To do this, put lemongrass in clusters in a liter jar, without tamping, and pour alcohol to the top. Put in a dark place for 2 weeks. After that, mix all 3 tinctures at the rate of: 1 tablespoon of tinctures from aspen bark and lemongrass per 100 g of redberry tincture (bugs). Take the resulting tincture of 20 g 3 times a day half an hour before meals (do not drink or eat!). Course - 3 months. Important: alcohol should not be consumed at this time. After treatment, it is recommended to do an ultrasound scan, the adenoma should decrease.

Redberries are an excellent diuretic. Krasnikaneeded for beriberi, gastritis with low acidity of gastric juice, has antiseptic, tonic properties, improves digestion and intestinal motility, helps the heart and blood vessels.

Herbal treatment with lemongrass for prostate adenoma

1 part lemongrass fruit

1 part black elderberry flowers

1 part immortelle flowers

1 part tansy flowers

1 part nettle herb

1 part flax herb

1 part herbcelandine

1 part yarrow herb

0.5 l water

Grind and mix 2 tablespoons of the collection, pour water, cook in a water bath for 10-15 minutes, cool and strain. The resulting broth should be drunk 3 times a day for half an hour before meals.

Immortelle treats diseases of the kidneys, bladder, liver, gallbladder, helps with gastroenterological problems.

Tansy has an antiseptic and antispasmodic effect, is used for liver diseases, intestinal diseases, as an antipyretic and diaphoretic.

Celandine is an amazing herb. It treats almost everything - diseases of the kidneys and urinary tract, skin diseases, diseases of the liver, gallbladder, nasopharynx and oral cavity, gastrointestinal tract, metabolism, good for allergies, hypertension, gout. Helps heal wounds due to its bactericidal properties, soothes, fights inflammation and viruses. But the herb is poisonous and should be used with care.

Lemongrass tea with herbs for the treatment of prostate adenoma

1 part lemongrass fruit

1 part linden flowers

1 part mint flowers

1 part hawthorn flowers

1 part thyme flowers

1 part flowers and leavessweet clover

1 part petalswhite and red rose

1 part cumin seeds

1 part blackcurrant leaves

1 part fireweed leaves (willow-herb)

1 cup boiling water

This collection can be drunk as tea, brewing one tablespoon of crushed collection in a glass of boiling water.

Thyme (Bogorodskayagrass) - relieves inflammation, spasms, disinfects, soothes, has an expectorant and analgesic effect.

Rose petals

The narrow-leaved fireweed is characterized by powerfulanti-inflammatory,
neurosis, is an antioxidant.

Lemongrass and hazel leaves for prostate treatment

1 teaspoon lemongrass fruit

1 tablespoon hazel leaves or bark

1 cup boiling water

Brew the chopped components with a glass of boiling water, simmer for 15 minutes, leave for 40 minutes, strain. Drink 1-2 tablespoons several times a day.

Lemongrass and seeds of 6 plantsfor the treatment of prostatitis

1 part dried lemongrass

1 part psyllium lanceolate seeds

1 part black onion seeds

1 part parsley seeds

1 part coriander seeds

1 part colza seeds

1 part seedscarrots

0.5 l boiling water

Grind 2 tablespoons of the mixture in a mortar, brew with boiling water and hold in a water bath for 30 minutes. Insist overnight and drink in the morning and evening 30 minutes before meals, 1 glass of decoction.

Psyllium seeds are often used as a diuretic and for impotence. In addition, psyllium has anti-inflammatory,hemostatic,

Parsley relieves difficult and painful urination in violation of the function of the prostate gland, improves digestion, is used for gastritis, gastric and duodenal ulcers.

coriander seeds

The colza was used in ancient Greece for male diseases. Also, colza is used as a diuretic, relieves fatigue.

Carrot seeds have long been used

in folk medicine for kidney stones, sexual weakness, and also as a diuretic.

Lemongrass and licorice for the treatment of prostatitis

2 teaspoons lemongrass fruit

1 tablespoon licorice root

0.5 l water

Pour the crushed ingredients with water and cook them for 10 minutes. After cooling, strain and take 30-50 ml before each meal.

Chapter 4 Lemongrass in Other Diseases

Lemongrass for diabetes

Both tincture, and decoction, and lemongrass fruit juice reduce the concentration of sugar in the blood. The usual course is one month. These herbal medicines are effective only in mild forms of diabetes; in severe types of the disease, they are used as an adjuvant.

Tincture

In diabetes, pharmacy tincture of lemongrass is useful. Take 20-40 drops in the morning and afternoon with water. You can make a tincture at home: pour ripe and dried lemongrass fruits with 70% alcohol (1:5), leave for 10 days. Take 20-30 drops 2 times a day in the morning and in the afternoon before meals.

Decoction

10 g drylemongrass fruits

1 cup hotwater

Pour lemongrass with water, boil for 15 minutes, strain and bring to the original volume. Take 1 tablespoon morning and afternoon.

Juice

Fresh juice of lemongrass berries is taken 1 tablespoon 2-3 times a day.

Cake

Experts believe that pomace from

lemongrass leaves reducesblood sugar concentration. The amount of cake should be small, and the dose is selected according to the sensations, but it should not be more than 3 tablespoons per day.

Lemongrass with mistletoe and asparagus for diabetes

The mixture is shown not only as an aid in the treatment of diabetes, but is also recommended for anemia, loss of strength.

30 g powder fromlemongrass fruits

150 g asparagus root powderlight

30 g mistletoe herb powder

some honey

Turn a mixture of powders with honey into pills and take 3-5 pieces 2-3 times a day.

To improve vision

Lemongrass is able to increase visual acuity with myopia,glaucoma and other eye diseases: the plant increases the sensitivity of the retina to light stimuli.

Schisandra berries to improve vision

10 g drylemongrass fruits

1 cup hotwater

Pour lemongrass with water, boil for 15 minutes, strain and bring to the original volume. Take 1 tablespoon morning and afternoon.

For vision problems, it is necessary to use fresh lemongrass fruits: no more than 2-5 fruits 2 times in the morning. You can also take seed powder 1 g 2 times a day.

Lemongrass seed powder

Schisandra seed powder is shown to enhance visual acuity and accelerate eye adaptation to darkness. It is taken 0.5-1 g 2-3 times a day half an hour before meals. The course is one month. Courses can be repeated 3-4 times a year. The powder is also good for improving metabolism.

Lemongrass, juniper, plantain, rosehip

1 tablespoon lemongrass berries

25 juniper berries

30 rose hips

1 tablespoon plantain herb

0.5 l water

Grind raw materials, pour water, boil for 20 minutes, strain. Drink 1/2 cup 3 times a day. The course is one month.

Schisandra for farsightedness

5 tablespoons lemongrass chinensis fruit

500 ml alcohol

Grind the fruits well, pour with alcohol, put for 10 days in a dark place, but not in the refrigerator, shake at least 1 time per day.

Strain, squeeze the fruit. Take tincture of 20 drops, dissolving in water, before meals 1-2 times a day.

Lemongrass seed tincture will also help improve eyesight - see the recipe in Chapter 2 "Schisandra Seed Tincture".

To regulate the functioning of the nervous system

Lemongrass has an excellent property to increase the reflex activity of the nervous system, enhancing positive reflexes and motor activity and without depleting nerve cells (unless, of course, there is an overdose in taking Schizandra preparations, which can result in insomnia, tachycardia, and a sharp increase in blood pressure) . Among adaptogens, this is the most powerful stimulator of excitation processes in the central nervous system. This was known in antiquity.

Adaptogens were known and used in antiquity, millennia 6–7 BC. Word

"adaptogen" - derived from the term "adaptation" (adaptation). Adaptogens adapt us to any adverse factors: cold, heat, oxygen deficiency, physical and mental overload. They help the patient recover faster after surgery, regulate the overall balance in the body, optimize brain function, increase intellectual productivity, reaction speed, and make learning and memorization processes more efficient. Moreover,adaptogens help muscles use energy more economically, improve protein synthesis, which in turn

– improves

our memory. Adaptogens perfectly strengthen the body as a whole, and they can strengthen it so much that it already copes with a number of diseases on its own or does not allow them at all. Adaptogens contain substances that have an anti-stress effect at the level of cellular metabolism. Most often, small doses of adaptogens inhibit nervous system, medium - tone up, large doses

– strongly

activate and excite. For adaptogens,in addition to lemongrass, include ginseng, leuzeasafflower-like (maral root), eleutherococcus prickly, rhodiola rosea (golden root), Manchurian aralia, zamaniha high.

Adaptogens are a treasure trove for athletes, knowledge workers, for those who want to lose weight. These drugs act quite effectively and quickly, but in no case should the dosage be exceeded, excess can lead to heart palpitations, increased pressure, etc. Adaptogens should not be used with strong arousal, hypertension and feverish conditions. It is not recommended to take them after dinner. And if you take adaptogens (most often they are used in the form of tinctures) to excite the nervous system in the morning, it will not be out of place to remind you that you should not use the same tincture for more than a month and a half, and in the evening it is desirable to calm the nervous system. For this, there are other tinctures: motherwort, valerian, Baikal skullcap. Take them to soothe 20-30 drops at night.

According to the strength of its activating effect on the body, lemongrass is not inferior to a number of doping drugs. Therefore, it is used most often for the treatment of asthenic and asthenodepressive conditions (psychasthenia, neurasthenia, traumatic cerebral palsy, atherosclerotic neurasthenia, reactive depression in patients with atherosclerosis).

Lemongrass works great for mental and physical overwork.

Do not use lemongrass for hysteria and insomnia.

If you take lemongrass once, it will act like a cup of coffee, but a little softer will increase and decrease arousal. If you take lemongrass for a week, your performance will increase markedly, sleep will improve, falling asleep and waking up will become easy, and sleep willdeep. The mood is harmonized. At first, it is recommended to take lemongrass in very small doses so as not to cause a powerful excitation of the body.

Lemongrass juice is very good for improving the functioning of the nervous system. It can be added 2 teaspoons in the morning to tea (how to make juice from lemongrass berries, see the second chapter: “Natural lemongrass juice”).

No less good in terms of effects is the infusion of lemongrass fruits (see recipe

in the second chapter: "Infusion of lemongrass berries").

You can use lemongrass essential oil (sold in a pharmacy): it helps to concentrate activity, improves memory, enhances stamina, stimulates metabolism, and is an excellent adaptogen.

Alcohol tincture of lemongrass is an excellent tool for regulating the processes of excitation and inhibition in the central nervous system.

To enhance inhibition, select the optimal dosage starting with 5-10 drops of alcohol tincture of magnolia vine. For gettingtonic and stimulating effect, you need to start with 10-15 drops. These are indicative doses. Exact doses need to be selected individually, empirically.

Alcohol tincture of lemongrass

This tincture is good for asthenia and nervous breakdown.

20 g ripe and dried lemongrass

100 ml 70% alcohol

Pour the berries of lemongrass with alcohol, insist for 10 days.

Take 20-30 drops 2 times a day, morning and afternoon 30 minutes before meals. The course of treatment is from 20 to 35 days.

With weakness, fatigue, drowsiness, decreased performance, depression and asthenic syndromes, tincture from the fruits of Chinese magnolia vine is drunk 2 times a day before meals for 20 drops. The same dose is indicated for increased psychophysical stress and when working in extreme conditions. In special cases, the dose can be increased to 35-40 drops.

Lemongrass and thyme for nervous disorders

1 teaspoon crushed lemongrass

1 teaspoon chopped thyme (thyme) herb

1 cup boiling water

Lemongrass fruit and thyme herbpour a glass of boiling water, insist, tightly closed and wrapped, 1 hour. Drink 1 tablespoon of infusion in the morning and evening. Infusion cook every day.

Lemongrass is a wonderful remedy for astheno-depressive syndrome, characterized by fatigue and irritable weakness.

An infusion of lemongrass leaves and stems will well relieve depression of the asthenic type. It is necessary to brew fresh or dried leaves and stems of lemongrass as tea at the rate of 1 teaspoon of crushed raw materials per 1 cup of boiling water.

Lemongrass, sage and elecampane for nervous disorders

2 g shootslemongrass

10 g sage herb

5 g elecampane roots

1 glass of water

Prepare a crushed mixture of lemongrass shoots, sage herb and elecampane roots, pour water, boil for 10-15 minutes and leave for 1 hour. Add cinnamon to taste. Drink during the day half an hour before meals or 4 hours after meals.

Lemongrass, mint, bearberry for neurasthenia

30 g mint leaves

10 g magnolia chinensis seeds

15 g bearberry leaves

2 glasseswater

Pour the crushed collection with boiling water and insist for 3 hours.Take 1 tablespoon 4 times a day. The course of taking the infusion is two weeks, then you need to take a break for one week.

Lemongrass essential oil in a mixture of oils for stress relief It is necessary to mix essential oils in an aroma lamp:

1 drop lemongrass

2 drops of lemon balm

2 drops bigardia

1 drop sage

1 drop chamomile

1 drop galbanum

Essential oil of lemongrassmixtures of oils for emotional tone These mixtures can not only be lit in aroma lamps, but also added to

bath.

It is necessary to mix the oils in the following proportions:

1 drop lemongrass

2 drops rosemary

2 drops of orange

1 drop of nutmeg

1 drop of damask rose

Lemongrass for women

Lemongrass is excellent for early toxicosis and lowering blood pressure in pregnant women, with asthenia after pathological childbirth and abdominal operations. It is also needed for menopause, which is not accompanied by either an increase or a decrease in blood pressure. To relieve menopausal syndrome - nervous tension, irritability, bad mood - it is recommended to drink an infusion or tincture of lemongrass berries.

To improve ovarian function and infertility

Helps to establish the work of the

ovaries alcohol tincture of magnolia vine. It is necessary to take 15 drops 2 times a day for 3 weeks. Recommended tincture and infertility.

With menopause, lemongrass essential oil and lemongrass tincture will help. The fact is that in the oil and tincture there are hormone-like substances that have a good effect on the body during menopausal changes in hormonal balance.

Lemongrass tones the smooth muscles of the uterus, therefore it is used in the treatment of a number of gynecological diseases, including female infertility, as an adjuvant in complex therapy.

Lemongrass with herbs for inflammation of the appendages

Such a collection has an antibacterial, anti-inflammatory, immunostimulating effect.

1 part lemongrass fruit

1 part lure roots

1 part ginseng roots

1 part plantain leaves

1 part leavescranberries

1 part St. John's wort

1 part fruitchestnut

0.5 l boiling water

Brew two tablespoons of chopped raw materials with boiling water. Infuse for 30 minutes, strain and take 150 ml 3 times a day before meals. The course of treatment is 1 month. Every day prepare a new infusion.

Chapter 5 Lemongrass for Skin

In dermatology, Schisandra chinensis preparations are used in the treatment of eczema, dermatitis, urticaria, and various skin diseases of unclear etiology (allergodermatosis, vasculitis, psoriasis, lichen planus, cystic, viral dermatosis, vitiligo, alopecia). At the same time, lemongrass helps as a wound healing agent that promotes the formation of young skin, as well as an immunostimulant and a drug that improves metabolic processes in the body. That is, for skin diseases, lemongrass is shown in anytypes (tea, infusion, decoction, tincture, juice, etc.) - it will strengthen the body.

Before starting treatment with lemongrass preparations for skin diseases, be sure to consult your doctor.

For eczema

For the treatment of eczema and inflammatory skin diseases, the following ointment is recommended: insist on the pulp of lemongrass fruit in water or alcohol, thicken at a temperature of 60-80 C, apply to the affected area.

For various skin diseases

Medical research in laboratories in different countries (USA, UK, France, China, Hong Kong, South Korea) have shown that ancient Chinese recipes are confirmed by modern science.

In particular, it has been proven that the best preparation for topical application and application towounds, dermatitis, eczema, psoriasis, trophic ulcers is an infusion of lemongrass seeds with simultaneous intake of seed powder inside.

Lemongrass infusion for external use:

1 teaspoon lemongrass seed powder

1 glass of water

Crush dry lemongrass seeds in a mortar. Store the powder in a cool dry place.

Pour 1 teaspoon of powder with a glass of boiling water, bring to a boil and immediately remove from heat. Cool down. Strain through a double cheesecloth, napkin or non-woven towel. Pour into a tightly closed jar or bottle and store in the refrigerator.

For minor skin lesions, apply to the wound or damaged areas with a cotton swab.

For chronic and complex wounds, it is better to make lotions and dressings: moisten a napkin or a piece of bandage in the infusion, apply to the wound, cover with cellophane film on top and secure with a bandage. You can change the bandage 2-3 times a day until complete healing. In difficult cases, after 3 weeks, you should pause for a week, then repeat the treatment.

Seed intake:

These procedures will be much more effective if the powder is taken orally at the same time. You can simply eat 1/3 teaspoon of lemongrass powder 2-3 times a day or take 1 tablespoon of the infusion 30-40 minutes before meals.

Warning:

With high blood pressure, angina attacks, and patients with epilepsy, Schisandra should not be taken orally. It is better for such patients to confine themselves only to the external use of lemongrass.

Lemongrass with herbs for eczema

1 part lemongrass fruit

1 partsage (leaves)

1 part plantain leaves

1 part leavesnettle

1 part wormwood (herb)

1 part yarrow herb

1 partHypericum

1 part juniper fruit

1.5 cups boiling water

1 liter of water

All components are mixed, 2

tablespoons of the crushed mixture are poured with boiling water, heated in a water bath for 10 minutes, infused for 20 minutes, filtered, the raw material is squeezed out, the resulting infusion is mixed with 1 liter of water. Drink 4 times a day for 1/2 cup 1 hour before meals.

Lemongrass and herbal collection for psoriasis

1 part lemongrass fruit

1 part herb string

1 part black elderberry flowers

1 part St. John's wort

1 part herbcelandine

1 part elecampane root

1 part calamus root

1 part leavescranberries

1 part horsetail herbfield

2 parts mint leavespeppery

1.5 cups boiling water

1 liter of water

All components are mixed, 2 tablespoons of the crushed mixture are poured with boiling water, heated in a water bath for 15 minutes,insist 20 minutes, filter, squeeze the raw materials and the resulting infusion is diluted in 1 liter of water. Drink 4 times a day for 1/2 cup 1 hour before meals.

Lemongrass and a variety of herbs for psoriasis

1 teaspoon lemongrass tincture

100 g elderberry flowers

100 g St. John's wort

100 g of celandine herb

100 g lingonberry leaves

one hundredg hop cones

100 g burdock root

1 tablespoon string juice

0.5 l boiling water

1.5pour tablespoons of crushed

collection with boiling water, cook under the lid for 5 minutes. Insist 30 minutes. Strain and add string juice and lemongrass tincture. Take half a cup 4 times a day one hour before meals.

Lemongrass shoots and 6 herbs

5 g shootslemongrass

5 g sage herb

2 g horsetail

2 g stinging nettle leaves

3 g violet tricolor herb

1 g parsley herb

3 g chicory herb

200 ml boiling water

Pour boiling water over 1 teaspoon of chopped collection, leave for 8-10 hours, strain, take 0.5 cup 3-4 times a day 30 minutes before meals for 1-2 months.

Herbal collection with lemongrass for dermatitis

5 g shootslemongrass

3 g herb tripartite

10 g wild strawberry leaves

10 g viburnum flowers

3 g fruitswild rose

200 ml boiling water

pour a teaspoon of the collection with boiling water, leave for 8-10 hours, strain, take 0.5 cups 3-4 times a day 30 minutes before meals for 1-2 months.

Lemongrass juice for allergic

With severe itching, the skin is rubbed with lemongrass juice.

Lemongrass essential oil is an anti-pediculosis agent, as well as an antidote.insect bites: eliminates itching, burning, swelling.

Lemongrass essential oil for fungal diseases of the skin of the feet

3 drops lemongrass essential oil

5 drops of tea tree essential oil

1 drop thyme essential oil

10 g vegetableoils

Mix essential oils with vegetable oils

Schisandra - home cosmetologist

In China, women have long used lemongrass juice as a rejuvenating drug. “Whoever drinks lemongrass juice,” says an ancient Chinese manuscript, “wrinkles are smoothed out, the skin becomes soft and supple, like a rose petal.”

Since I have been using lemongrass in various forms for a long time, I could not help but notice how wonderfully lemongrass also affects my skin: the skin becomes younger and less flabby due to the fact that its protective properties improve, irritation is removed, fine wrinkles are smoothed out. This is largely due to the presence of essential fatty acids, especially linolenic acid, in lemongrass seeds. If the body does not have enough of them, the skin can become dry, begin to peel off, and be irritated.

Lemongrass enhances the regeneration and renewal of skin cells, and also tones them.

In modern cosmetology, lemongrass extract and essential oil are used. Face masks with the addition of lemongrass, hair balms, tonic creams for the face and for skin care around the eyes are produced. But you can make your own cosmetics using lemongrass preparations. Suitable for this and berries, and leaves, and bark, and young shoots of the plant.

Toning mask for all skin

2 tablespoons sour cream

2 drops alcohol tincture of lemongrass

1 tablespoon curd

Mix all ingredients. Apply to the face for 10 minutes, then rinse with a swab dipped in lemongrass tea or warm water. Wash off with cool water.

Moisturizing mask for all skin types

2 tablespoons dried lemongrass berries

1 cup boiling water

2 teaspoons honey

Crush lemongrass berries in a mortar, pour boiling water in an enamel saucepan, bring to a boil, reduce heat, boil for 15 minutes, cool, strain. Add honey, soak gauze with the mixture and apply on face, neck, décolleté for 15 minutes. Then wash with water at room temperature.

Infusion of lemongrass against wrinkles

An infusion of the fruit can be used to wipe

It is necessary to pour 10 g of lemongrass fruits with a glass of boiling water, insist20 minutes and strain.

Refreshing lotion for oily skin

2 tablespoons chopped fresh lemongrass

0.5 l vodka

1 tablespoon glycerin

It is necessary to fill the lemongrass berries with vodka and leave for a week in a dark place, then strain and squeeze the berries. Add glycerin. Before use, the tincture should be diluted with water in a ratio of 1: 3 and wipe the skin of the face in the morning and evening.

Lemongrass ice with herbs for oily and combination skin

1 part lemongrass fruit

1 part chamomile flowers

1 part marigold flowers

1 part celandine

500 ml boiling water

pour tablespoons of crushed collection with boiling water, leave for 2 hours, then let cool, strain, pour into ice molds and freeze. Wash your face in the evening.

Lemongrass ice with juices for oily and combination skin

1 teaspoon juice mixture of lemongrass, lingonberry and blueberry

1 cup boiledwater

Add a mixture of juices to a glass of boiled water. Pour the resulting liquid into ice molds and place in the freezer.

Contraindications for

Wiping the skin of the face with ice cubes is not recommended in winter, before going out, with a tendency to colds, and also if the skin is dehydrated and irritated or has pronounced dilated capillaries.

Mask for dry skin

1 teaspoon chopped fresh lemongrass

1 tablespoon full fat sour cream(25%)

some milk (2.5-3.2%)

Mix lemongrass fruits with sour cream and apply on the face for 10 minutes, then wash off the mask with milk.

For porous skin

To narrow the pores, you need to wipe the skin in the morning and evening with lemongrass oil.

Lemongrass oil, due to its astringent properties, fights against excessive oiliness of the skin, tightens pores, dilates blood vessels, helps reduce wrinkles. Since the essential oil of magnolia vine is not produced industrially, a mixture of fatty and essential oils of lemongrass is sold in pharmacies, and this mixture can often be called essential oil. But in any case, no matter how this oil is called, it has a very good effect on the skin.

In addition to lemongrass, essential oils of bergamot, juniper, and chamomile are distinguished by their ability to narrow pores. You can add 1-2 drops of these oils to any tonic, mask or cream.

Important: essential oils should not be used by pregnant women and epileptics.

Mask with essential oil of lemongrass to narrow the pores

2 drops lemongrass essential oil

2 drops bergamot (juniper, chamomile) essential oil

2 teaspoons of jojoba oil

2 teaspoons sweet almond oil

Mix essential and fatty oils. Every evening, apply the mixture on cleansed skin of the face, after 5-7 minutes, remove the excess oil that has not been absorbed with a paper towel.

Enrichment of the cream with lemongrass essential oil - for oily porous skin

10 ml cream

1 drop lemongrass essential oil

2 drops of chamomile essential oil

1 drop essential oilpines

Mix the ingredients and use as a regular face cream.

Variety of uses of lemongrass essential oil.

In aroma lamps: 2-4 drops per 15 m2.

For massage: 3-4 drops per 15 g of transport oil.

To enrich cosmetic preparations: 3 drops per 15 g of base.

To tighten cratered pores: Mix 7 drops of lemongrass oil with 10 drops of wheat germ oil. Apply with an applicator to porous areas and leave for 5-7 minutes, then wash with vegetable soap, rinse your face with rosewood water and apply a moisturizer or jojoba oil with chamomile essential oil - 4 drops per 15 g of base. The procedure should be repeated no more than 1 time in 3 days, the number of procedures is 10–20.

Disinfection of items: 10 drops of lemongrass oil in a glass of water. Treat the surface with a cloth or sponge soaked in this solution.

Internal use: 1 drop with honey, jam, butter, in a bread "pill" 2 times a day (do not take before bedtime!). Drink juice, tea, kefir.

Contraindications.Do not use during pregnancy. Do not apply to dry, sensitive areas of the skin. Do not use for more than 14 days continuously. It is necessary to test the aroma for individual tolerance.

Washing lotion for oily porous skin

3 drops lemongrass essential oil

100 ml water

Dissolve the oil in water and use the lotion to wash. Steam bath for the face with oily porous skin

1 drop lemongrass essential oil

2 drops bergamot essential oil

0.5 l water

Prepare a steam bath from these components and steam your face for 10 minutes.

Lemongrass scrub

10 drops lemongrass essential oil

5 drops of geranium essential oil

5 drops fennel essential oil

2 teaspoons sweet almond oil

4 tablespoons of sugar

Mix all oils with sugar and use as a scrub.

How to choose essential oils.

High-quality essential oil has a transparent and uniform consistency. If you drop the oil on a piece of paper, then after it evaporates there is no greasy stain left. It is better to buy essential oils from well-known companies that specialize in this product. Quality oils are not cheap, as they are expensive to manufacture. It is necessary to take the oil of those companies that indicate in the accompanying instructions both the Latin names of the plants from which the oil was produced and the date of production. It is not necessary to buy essential oils in vials with rubber stoppers or in plastic capsules (essential oils can corrode rubber and plastic), as well as in light glass vials (light can negatively affect their quality). Essential oils evaporate easily and are sensitive to light, so they should be stored in the dark, in a cool place, hermetically sealed in dark glass vials.

Hair conditioner

This tool strengthens the hair roots and stimulates their growth.

1 tablespoon of a mixture of crushed fresh leaves, small twigs and fruits

0.5 l boiling water

Pour a mixture of crushed fresh leaves, small twigs and fruits with boiling water, insist in a thermos for 2-3 hours, strain and squeeze out the raw materials. Use as a final rinse after shampooing.

If your hair falls out, you can use the experience of Japanese women: many centuries ago, they rubbed into hair to restore hair.scalp thick juice from under the bark of lemongrass creeper.

If you rinse your hair with a decoction of lemongrass fruits or leavesafter washing, they will grow better, be silky and shiny.

"Rejuvenating" bath

This bath tones and rejuvenates the skin and the entire body.

4 tablespoons chopped dried lemongrass leaves

1 liter of boiling water

Pour the leaves with boiling water,

leave for 1 hour, strain, add to the bath at a temperature of 37 C. Take 15 minutes.

If you have prepared dry lemongrass leaves and have lain with you for more than two years, do not throw them away. It is better to put the leaves in a nylon bag and lower it into the water when taking a bath. The skin will look younger.

Chapter 6 How to grow lemongrass in the country

Schisandra chinensis grows successfully in my dacha in the Smolensk region. If you set out to grow this healing plant on your site, I am sure that you will succeed, as I did.

Among the vines, only lemongrass - the most frost-resistant and early ripening vine - climbed so far north - up to Karelia.

Of course, lemongrass is a little more capricious than sea buckthorn, which is so common in our country, but an amateur summer resident is quite capable of coping with his whims.

At my dacha, lemongrass blooms in late May - very early June. This is a liana up to 10 m long or more. It spirals - clockwise -wraps around nearby trees and bushes. The roots of the creeper are shallow - at a depth of up to 30 cm and are highly branched.

Lemongrass has waxy, fragrant, pinkish or creamy white, bell-shaped flowers. The berries of lemongrass are first light green, then white, pink and then become red-orange tones, reminiscent of the color of Russian mountain ash, and the shape is a branch of red currant, only the berries are not on the stalks, but are attached directly to the branch - that is, they look like elongated bunches. They ripen in September, they can hang all winter on a bush and not crumble.

On an adult bush (schisandra begins to actively bear fruit by about 7 years of age), 4-5 kg of berries can grow in the best years. Picked berries must be processed immediately, as they deteriorate rather quickly - they are covered with a white moldy coating. Berries have one or two seeds.

Schisandra seeds are yellow-orange in color, with a smooth, shiny surface, covered with a dense shell, having a bitter-burning taste.

The first 3-5 years, lemongrass grows very slowly, but then picks up growth. It is better not to transplant lemongrass bushes. Lemongrass is not love pests, which is very good. Fungal diseases practically do not appear outwardly, except that in wet and cold weather, you can notice a fungal coating on fading leaves. adult bushesquite unpretentious, require minimal care, for example, watering in hot and dry summers; for the winter in central Russia, lemongrass can not be covered.

I got my few lemongrass bushes from seeds that relatives sent me from the Khabarovsk Territory.

It is in the Far East (Khabarovsk and Primorsky Territories, Amur and Sakhalin Regions) that Chinese magnolia vine grows in natural conditions. This plant is a relic: it survived the ice age and survived! Like 25 million years ago, in the Far Eastern forests, lemongrass densely wraps around shrubs and climbs tall trees. The main thickets of lemongrass are located in coniferous-deciduous forests of the Manchurian type. In the mountains above 500–600 m above sea level, lemongrass is not found. He loves optimally lit forests, actively bears fruit along river valleys, on roadsides, on edges, old clearings, where there is quite a lot of light, and there are also insects - pollinators of flowers. Now in Europe and America they have stopped looking at lemongrass as an exclusively ornamental plant called "winding magnolia",

Where is the best place to plant lemongrass at their summer cottage

The best place to plant is an elevated part of the site with good drainage, protected from cold winds and dry winds. Lemongrass is best suited for light penumbra, when the roots and lower part of the stems are shaded, and the upper branches are illuminated by the sun.

Since lemongrass looks very beautiful, it's a good idea to plant it near the facades of summer cottages, preferably on the western or southwestern side, as well as along garden paths, hedges, arches, arbors, etc. Delicate green leaves hang from thin vines, shine through the sun and create a unique openwork ligature. The distance between plants in a row when planting should be at least 1–1.5 m.

Lemongrass is planted in a permanent place in the garden at 2-3 years of age, it is better to plant in the spring. All operations associated with planting must be done quickly so that the roots of the seedling do not dry out. Plant at the same depth at which the plant grew before.

Lemongrass is not covered for the winter.

Soil and top dressing

Lemongrass, like many forest and taiga plants, loves light, loose and fertile soil, moist enough, but without groundwater stagnation and waterlogging. Such soil contributes to good winter hardiness of the plant. Schisandra drought resistance is low; in hot and dry summers, the soil must be watered periodically. It must be remembered that lemongrass does not tolerate not only overdrying of the soil, but also waterlogging. The roots of lemongrass lie shallow, so the soil should be loose, fertilized with humus; leafy is better. And it is categorically impossible to introduce unripe manure into the soil. During the growing season, you need to do several weeding and fine loosening of the soil. In addition, during the growing season, you need to add loose earth to the roots, make top dressing with organic and mineral fertilizers.

Organic fertilizers are pet manure, compost, bird droppings.

The most commonly used mineral fertilizers: nitrogen - ammonium nitrate, ammonium sulfate, phosphorus - superphosphate and potash - potassium sulfate, potassium salt, wood ash.

Lemongrass lovesnitrogen, superphosphate, potassium chloride, ordinary ash.

Good drainage is very important.

In the first two years, lemongrass grows very slowly. care at this time

- surface loosening of the soil, weeding, watering. In dry hot weather in the morning and evening, lemongrass needs to be sprayed with water, and the soil needs to be mulched.

Mulch is any material that covers

soil from above. Mulch retains moisture, protects the soil from temperature changes, keeps cool, conducts air, and prevents the destruction of soil structure. Usually, the soil under the lemongrass bushes is mulched with leafy humus.

After two years after planting, you need to feed the plants with organic and mineral fertilizers. In the spring, before bud break, 50 g of nitrophosphate per 1 m2 is applied under the creepers, the soil around them is loosened shallowly and mulched with humus; in autumn, 60 g of superphosphate and 30–40 g of potash fertilizers per 1 m2 are applied.

pruning lemongrass

Lemongrass tends to give a lot of shoots. At 3-4 years of life, it is advisable to cut the bush: remove extra shoots, leaving a few of the best. This will give the bush the opportunity to grow rapidly. If the bush is heavily thickened, you will not see the harvest. Schisandra chinensis flowers are wind pollinated. In order for pollen from a male flower to get to a female one, it is necessary that it does not get stuck in thick leaves. Also, Schisandra's male flowers tend to be in the lower tier of the bush, so the pollen must be blown up by the wind! Without pruning, pollination simply will not take place!

Pruning must be done carefully so

as not to damage the remaining branches. Pruning is preferable in late autumn, since pruning in spring causes abundant sap production, and it weakens the bush.

Reproduction of lemongrass

In the wild, lemongrass can be propagated by seeds and vegetatively. Cultivated lemongrass is most often propagated by seeds. This takes more time than the vegetative propagation method, but is more effective for future fruiting. Use freshly harvested seeds or those that have been stored dry for less than a year and have been stratified. Seed stratification is a method of pre-sowing preparation to accelerate germination after sowing.

The plant is also propagated vegetatively (rhizome shoots, layering and cuttings). Seeds can be sown both in autumn and spring. But since the seeds lose their germination after about six months, it is better to sow them in the fall in boxes or in open ground. During the winter, natural stratification of seeds will take place, and friendly shoots will appear. It is important to know that magnolia vine quite often has empty seeds: at the same time, outwardly normal seeds do not have an embryo. So in good conditions, about 2/3 of the seeds germinate.

This is how I worked with my seeds. In the autumn, she sowed the seeds in a long box, which she left for the winter on the site, covered with leaves and dry plants, and in the winter she buried them in the snow. The box before germination can be covered with film or glass.

In May, shoots appeared, I moved the box to a place so that at noon it was exposed to scattered sunlight, after about a month it was possible to move the box to a completely open place. Several times I fed the plants with mineral fertilizers and watered moderately.

In autumn, lemongrass plants were already up to 10 cm tall. They wintered in the same way as in the first winter - in a box under the snow. And in the spring Itransplanted plants - with a clod of earth around the roots - to an open place on the site. And by autumn they had already risen by 80-90 centimeters. In the fourth year after planting, lemongrass bushes bloomed, and in the fall I harvested the first crop.

How to Stratify Seeds

Before spring sowing, seeds can be stratified as follows:

Soak the seeds for 4 days in water, change the waterdaily.

Wrap the seeds in a nylon bag and bury them in moist - preferably river and calcined in the oven - sand in a wooden box. Cover the top of the box with a sheet of filter paper and pour over.

The optimum stratification temperature is 18-20 °C. Once a week, the seeds need to be aired: dig a bag of sand, open for 10 minutes and mix. Then place it back in the bag and rinse under running water, squeeze a little and bury it in the sand again. It is necessary to ensure that the sand in the box does not dry out.

After a month, move the box to the cold - deep under the snow and keep it there for another month.

Then place the seed box in a room with a temperature of no more than 10 C (in the basement).

Seedlings should appear in about three weeks.

Seeds should be sown in boxes with a mixture of soil, peat and river sand in a ratio of 1:2:1 to a depth of 0.5 cm, water and then monitor the soil moisture, preventing it from drying out.

When 3-4 leaves appear,

seedlings can be sown on ridges or in a cold greenhouse. They put them in rows.

After sowing, plants need to be shaded and watered.

Seedlings at the age of one year have a height of up to 6 cm, 7-9 leaves and a root system up to 12 cm long.

How to propagate lemongrass

The vegetative propagation method is good for propagating high-yielding bushes.

For propagation by layering in autumn or early spring, you need to dig grooves 15-20 cm deep around the bush, bend the branch to the bottom of the groove, pin it with wooden pegs to the soil, cover it with earth, and leave the top of the shoot on the soil surface. It's best to do it in the spring. Layers need to be watered regularly. Six months later, the vine sprinkled with earth will take root, and after another year and a half it will be possible to carefully separate the layering from the bush with a pruner, dig it up and transplant it to the chosen place.

When propagating with green cuttings, three factors must be borne in mind: the timing of cutting cuttings, the age of the mother bush, and treatment with growth stimulants. Shoots should be cut before or during flowering (May - early June), because after flowering they quickly become woody, which will result in poor rooting of the cuttings. Schizandra practically does not take root with winter woody cuttings. The younger the mother plant, the better the rooting occurs. It is better to cut cuttings from two to three year old bushes. Cuttings are cut 4–8 cm long with two or three nodes from shoots growing in the middle and lower parts of the bush. The lower cut should be made 3–5 mm below the kidney, the upper cut 2–4 mm above it. Cuttings should be treated with a solution of heteroauxin (100 mg per 1 liter of water), kept in solution for about a day, this will speed up rooting.

It is desirable to root green cuttings in a greenhouse filled with light and fertile soil, in a layer of sand 7–10 cm deep. The distance between cuttings in a row is about 7 cm, between rows - 10 cm, planting depth - 2–3 cm. Cuttings are watered and covered film or glass. On a hot day, you need to slightly open the film or glass on the leeward side.

In the early days, it is

recommended to spray the seedlings several times a day with water from a spray bottle.

It is better to plant seedlings in the spring. Roots should not be damaged or dry. You cannot cut them. To plant seedlings, you need to dig holes 70 cm deep and 50–60 cm wide at a distance of one and a half meters from each other, pour up to 10 cm on the bottom of river pebbles for good drainage (this is especially important for loams!). On the pour pebbles with river sand with a layer of up to 5 cm, on the sand - forest soil mixed with leafy humus, sand, mineral fertilizer (taken in equal parts) and three glasses of a glass of wood ash. For better pollination, and hence fruiting, you need to plant 2-3 seedlings in each hole, 3-5 cm deeper than they grew before transplanting. The roots must be carefully and carefully straightened and sprinkled with earth. After planting, and then as it dries up, it is recommended to moderately water the soil and mulch it with well-rotted manure with a layer of 2–3 cm. 15 kg of sand.

It is necessary to plant at least two seedlings half a meter apart from each other, which are taken from different places - while the vines will contain different varietal characteristics, which will have a beneficial effect on the harvest.

If lemongrass is propagated by basal shoots, it starts growing well in the second year, and the crop can be obtained in the fourth year after planting. This is a good way to propagate lemongrass, not very troublesome. Root shoots usually come to the surface of the soil, since the root system of the plant is not deep in the ground. On theone rhizome usually has several shoots. In spring or autumn, it is easy to separate them from the main bush and simply plant them as a separate bush.

How to care for adult vines

With the onset of fruiting, lemongrass no longer needs to be fed. It is enough to mulch in autumn - with leaves in a layer of 15–20 cm or with compost in a layer of 5 cm.

support for lemongrass

Support is an important condition for the upbringing and maintenance of the vine. Such a support is made for a long time, since lemongrass is very difficult to transfer to another support - its branches are strongly intertwined. In addition, lemongrass can grow and bear fruit in one place for a good half century, or even more. Interestingly, lemongrass vines twist only clockwise. They have very flexible and elastic shoots.

Poles were made from old metal pipes 2.5 m high in the country house, and between them a wire 5 mm thick was stretched in three rows. The bottom row was placed at a height of 0.5 m from the soil surface, the next row was placed 1 m later, and the third row was placed along the top of the support. And vertically, you can stretch the same wire at a distance of 30 cm between vertical rows. Or you can - an old electrical cord, twine. According to these devices, lemongrass will perfectly grow up.

If lemongrass is planted near the house, the support can be made in the form of a ladder that rises to the roof.

On a vertical support, lemongrass can rise to a height of up to10 m

Lemongrass perfectly decorates your site, you can dream up and make the support decorative too (or use the wall of the gazebo, arch, etc. to add decorativeness).

It is important to tie lemongrass to the supports on time, otherwise its abundant rhizomatous shoots will simply spread along the ground, and lemongrass will not bear fruit. As soon as lemongrass is tied to a support, it can produce a crop next year. The harvest from an adult bush (which is more than 6-7 years old) is about 3 kg of berries, but you need to remember that lemongrass does not bear fruit every year, but every 2-3 years.

Berries are located mainly at a height of more than 2.5 m, where the female flowers are most often found.

Harvesting lemongrass

Ripe fruits hang on the bush usually for about a month. Then they need to be collected with brushes and dried. I do it this way: I lay it out on the dachatable paper and put bunches of lemongrass on them. Be sure to dry in the shade. Paper needs to be changed from time to time. When the berries are dry, you need to fold the brushes into paper bags or cloth bags. Leaves are harvested during flowering, shoots - in the spring.

If, when harvesting lemongrass, you remove the seeds from the fruit, do not throw them away, but wash, dry and grind in a coffee grinder to a powder. Store the powder in tightly closed jars. Dried leaves can also be passed through a coffee grinder. To maintain a good tone, you will need both the one and the other powder - there are many recipes! Leaves are usually removed and dried during flowering.Dry leaves can be stored in cardboard boxes or glass jars with lids. For two years, they retain their medicinal properties

Lemongrass diseases

Lemongrass is not very susceptible to fungal and other diseases, but nevertheless, for prevention, you need to remove fallen leaves from under the bushes in the fall, and spray the leaves with 1% Bordeaux mixture in the spring.

Bordeaux liquid: a mixture of a solution of copper sulphate with milk of lime. It is necessary to dissolve copper sulphate and lime milk separately in water, then pour the copper sulphate solution in a thin stream into the lime solution and mix well. The mixture should be blue.

The most general rules for growing lemongrasscan be

summed up in several points:

plant in a shaded place on slightly acidic soil rich in organic fertilizers;

in the second year, tie to a support;

protect from ground and high water, the soil should

do not dig or loosen deep soil around magnolia vine;

water moderately.

www.ingramcontent.com/pod-product-compliance
Ingram Content Group UK Ltd.
Pitfield, Milton Keynes, MK11 3LW, UK
UKHW021937190726
13853UKWH00004B/1501

9 798417 968778